The Opposite of Burnout

5 Career Strategies to Feel Valued, Be Heard, and Make a Difference

CRISIS EDITION 2020

Liz Garrett

ISBN: 9798560172640

Cover design by: Liz Garrett

Printed in the United States of America

E.A., this is for you! You were right.
I should have listened sooner.

Table of Contents

Acknowledgments

To the many teachers whose concepts wove into the very fiber of my being, "thank you" is not enough. You saved me. This includes David Allen, Joseph Campbell, Jack Canfield, Edgar Cayce, Deepak Chopra, Stephen Covey, Wayne Dyer, Byron Katie, Jack Kornfield, Eckhart Tolle, Ken Wilbur, His Holiness the Dalai Lama, and many, many more. Your willingness to do the hard work of standing in your truth for the benefit of others, matters. With this book, I hope to pay it forward.

My deepest, heartfelt gratitude goes to Chris, who keeps me pointed toward my highest purpose, even when I can't see the way.

The path to this place has been long and convoluted. Every step was necessary. To the bad bosses and people left behind I owe a thank you and an apology. I couldn't give you my best, for that was yet to come. Thank you for helping me get there.

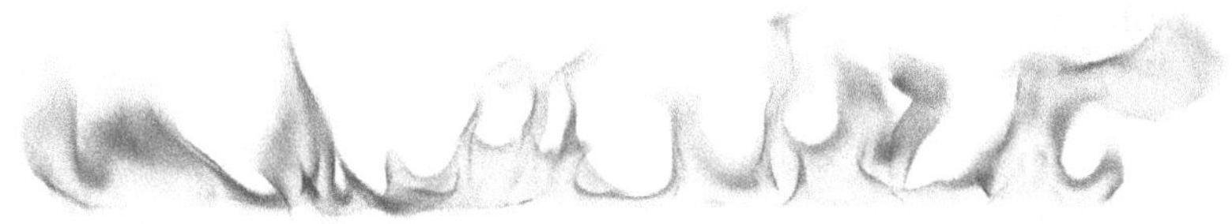

It Begins

IMAGINE A SEASONED LOG SUSPENDED above a dying fire. The embers below glow brilliant red, a coal heart: previous logs converted to carbon. The flames have died out. For the fire to be kept burning, to provide warmth and light to those who need it, it must have a constant source of fuel.

We can feed the log to the fire, energizing it in a flash of brilliance that serves many. The log will be consumed in the process. Maybe this is okay. Maybe it isn't.

There are other uses for the log. It can be used to build shelter, or a playground for children, or a pier out to a still lake. If we intercede early enough, the log could remain a living tree, preserving its potential for a future opportunity, or to serve its purpose as protection for the wild and shade for the weary.

What does the log want? Nobody asks it.

Until you decide otherwise, you are the log: a fuel source to be depleted for the communal fire. Your potential was recognized and harvested while you were still green, before you could weigh in on the choice. Very likely, you had test scores on the right end of a bell curve, and were directed down a path that, no doubt, opened doors, created opportunity, provided for you and your loved ones, and could consume you in the process. It's good work, but not necessarily fulfilling. Maybe your dreams, hopes and desires, recognized or not, have been suppressed to a persistent form of heartburn. You see yourself becoming increasingly cynical. You are dogged by unexplained exhaustion. Despite your resources, you feel stuck and strangely powerless. You are on your way to a coal heart.

This is your chance to jump out of the fire.

The Opposite of Burnout

When you push yourself all week to reach a goal or deadline and then, on Saturday, are too tired to push your child on a swing, that's burnout.

When you begin your week in deficit—not enough sleep, energy, passion, or interest in life—yet push yourself for full bore productivity, that's burnout.

When the spectrum of anger (which spans annoyance through rage) is your go-to emotion, day after day, that's burnout.

Or, when you build your life on a foundation of wishes, keeping your head down and blinders on in the name of work, until the first mean wind of life brings it all down like a house of cards, that's burnout. That's what happened to me. To avoid facing what wasn't right in my life, I worked harder, ignoring red flags, until a health emergency made everything else unsustainable. I burned out. I left a marriage, a job—no—a career. The cost was enormous: relationships, salary, years of career advancement, all gone. I was back to a beginning.

I want to spare you that outcome. I want the opposite for you.

What's the opposite of burnout? That's the beauty—you get to decide! It's your career, your life—if you don't decide its direction, who will?

This little book can help you figure that out, plus give you practical tools and actionable ideas to keep you on track for a meaningful, sustainable and lucrative career. Information is cool, but does nothing to improve your life. What you DO with the information makes a difference. This book emphasizes action.

The Slippery Slope of Burnout

There are reasons why certain professionals get hit hard by burnout (✓ Check off factors that apply):

- ☐ You studied hard in a challenging curriculum.
- ☐ You receive recognition: licensing, social status, family pride.
- ☐ You've never seriously considered alternatives.
- ☐ You feel the weight of your work. Your projects impact the future of society, but are mostly out of your control.
- ☐ Your work gets caught in the crush between "too much" and "not enough."
- ☐ Because you've invested so much, you can't just quit and walk away, especially if you are trapped by inertia, finances or lack of transferrable skills.

The modern work-style has eroded the quality of our personal lives. The digital invasion of home, blurring of work hours, and travel on weekends and holidays challenge life/work balance. People don't take vacations, or vacations are violated by phone and email. People don't feel safe taking personal time for self or family. Companies, pressured by competition and profit demands, may create fertile ground for burnout. ✓ Check off burnout factors existing in your workplace:

- [ ] Chronic overload: understaffing, workload issues;
- [ ] Cultural unfairness: favoritism, privilege, "the rules don't apply" to all equally, pay discrepancies;
- [ ] Conflicting values: company stated values are not followed by leadership; employee and company values are not in alignment;
- [ ] Constraints: employees lack autonomy and control, they feel unappreciated or disrespected, that their time is wasted, their requests denied;
- [ ] Cultural breakdown: no team spirit, no cohesion, no recognition of accomplishments, no celebration of success.

Psychologists Herbert Freudenberger, who coined the phrase "burnout" in 1974, and Gail North have identified 12 phases of burnout. These can occur in any order. ✓ Which do you see in you?

- [ ] The Compulsion to Prove Yourself – this looks like strong ambition
- [ ] Working Harder – doubling down to prove your value
- [ ] Neglecting Your Needs – work comes before eating, sleeping, and socializing
- [ ] Displacement of Conflicts – becoming aware that there is a problem, and blaming it on others
- [ ] Revision of Values – increasing isolation, conflict avoidance and denial of needs because the job is now the top priority
- [ ] Denial of Emerging Problems – marked by intolerance, aggression, sarcasm and avoidance of social contact
- [ ] Withdrawal – efforts to minimize contact, possible increase in drugs or alcohol, feelings of hopelessness
- [ ] Obvious Behavioral Changes – people are noticing and commenting on the ways you've changed
- [ ] Depersonalization – life becomes a series of mechanical functions with no thoughts, hopes or specific plans for the future
- [ ] Inner Emptiness – a gnawing sense of emptiness causes you to seek overeating, sex, alcohol, or drugs

- ☐ Depression – signs of clinical depression include exhaustion, hopelessness, indifference and, possibly, suicidal thoughts
- ☐ Full Burnout Syndrome – physical and mental collapse necessitating immediate medical attention.

✎ Make a T-chart:

Writing with pen on paper to maximize right-brain engagement, allow your thoughts to flow:

What's broken at work?	What's working at work?

There is no way around it. Achieving goals requires discipline and commitment. Everything else is an excuse. You already know this. Here's what may be new to you: you must direct that *same* discipline and commitment toward the care of yourself. You must have a strategy for career sustainability.

Your Strategy to Avoid Burnout

Congratulations! Your education and experience have served you well. Look how far you've come! However, education and experience are just your ante into the game. They are expected. Now that you're in, it's time to play to win. You need a game plan. You know "working harder and harder" is not a sustainable strategy. Instead, learn from professionals whose work makes them excited to get out of bed each day, who end the day satisfied with their accomplishments, who enjoy deep relationships, rich experiences, and unending abundance while making significant contribution to the world. These people have made a conscious choice and tenacious commitment to develop their gifts and talents using the strategies collected here.

This book covers the <u>5 Essential Strategies of Career Sustainability</u>:

1. **Self-Management**: The 5 Non-Negotiables—sleep, nutrition, physical activity, stress management, positive mindset—lay the foundation for success.
2. **Personal Branding**: Get clear on your strengths, how you want to be viewed and treated by others, and what you want to accomplish in this life.
3. **Mindful Organization:** What you do with your time, space and tasks either supports or impedes your success.
4. **Smart Communication:** Develop skills to convey information so that others are motivated and inspired to support your desired outcomes.
5. **Asset Protection:** Carpenters respect their hammer. Truckers maintain their semis. You need to protect and develop your best tool: your brain.

Stock Your Tool Chest

Chances are, you have some sort of toolset in your home. Maybe it's a shiny red, rolling cabinet with drawers, doors and a lift-up top. Or, maybe it's a drawer in your kitchen with a hammer and a screwdriver. Whatever it is, it is there, unused much of the time, but indispensable when you need it.

Take the same approach to avoiding burnout. Build an awesome tool chest. Then, use your tools. Rely on them every day for the rest of your life. This book has one purpose: to provide a variety of proven tools, hacks and habits you can use to beat burnout. It is FULL of tools: some you'll love, some you won't care for, some you'll need now, some you'll need later. And you will need them. Beating burnout is a continual, lifelong effort. Beating burnout is a lifestyle.

This book is one of your tools. It is small so that you can tuck it into your pocket, purse, tote, briefcase, or PLANNER. Dog-ear it, mark it up, make it your quick reference when you need it. download your collateral resources at https://LizGarrett.com/opposite/

An **organizing system** is one of the essential tools for keeping you focused on your priorities throughout the day. Assemble a system that feels good to you so you are attracted to using it. Keep it fresh—change styles, content and features as your preferences and needs change. Make it fun!

- Your system serves as a COLLECTION point for notes, ideas, and tasks, which you later process into your organizational system.
- Your system contains quick REFERENCES and LISTS that point you back to task or lift you when you slide.
- Your system holds your SUCCESS PLAN for today.
- Your system keeps your VISION and GOALS in front of you, reminding you of your strong "Why" when you must make moment-by-moment tough choices.
- Your system is your TOUCHSTONE reminder that you have a bigger purpose than the task at hand.
- Your system may or may not contain a CALENDAR, since digital management of your schedule has many benefits.
- Also, a system may or may not be a physical BINDER or PLANNER, since digital notebooks like OneNote and EverNote offer suitable alternatives. An effective system is dynamic, ever-evolving, and engaging.

This book supports you in developing:

▤ **Lists** – The wheel was a great invention, probably one of the all-time best. Don't keep reinventing it. Think something through once, write it down, and reference it as needed. Don't use brain capacity for storage. See a list of lists you might want to create at www.LizGarrett.com/opposite

⏻ **Habits/hacks** – Successful people know: habits can make or break you. Learn to leverage the power of effective habits. Take advantage of your brain's "autopilot" feature.

✍ **Processes/exercises** – These activities expedite decision making and facilitate deeper understanding so you can take action quickly: T-charts, mind maps, decision trees, etc.

◎ **Structures** – Use physical devices or symbols to keep you on track or to build in accountability. Examples include: screen saver message, wall chart for tracking, sticky notes, vision board, particular clothing, particular color, symbols, essential oils, theme song, deadlines that involve other people.

✓ **Check-offs** – Quickly and objectively assess your current situation.

AVOID OVERWHELM. This book condenses information and practices from many experts and sources. With its focus on IMPLEMENTATION, it contains more actions than any person could ever take over their entire career. Don't even try. The most effective way to make progress with this book is to implement ideas that carry a charge—interest you, intrigue you, excite you—*immediately*. Gain fast traction. Get results. See what works and what doesn't, and then. make adjustments. Revisit this book regularly.

Self Coaching: Get Started

Pause here. Before grabbing that planner and getting your systems in place, spend some time with this question:

♦♦♦

This is an action-oriented book. Make it yours. Mark it up. Carry it with you. Try various tools in various situations. Refer back as you and/or your situations change.

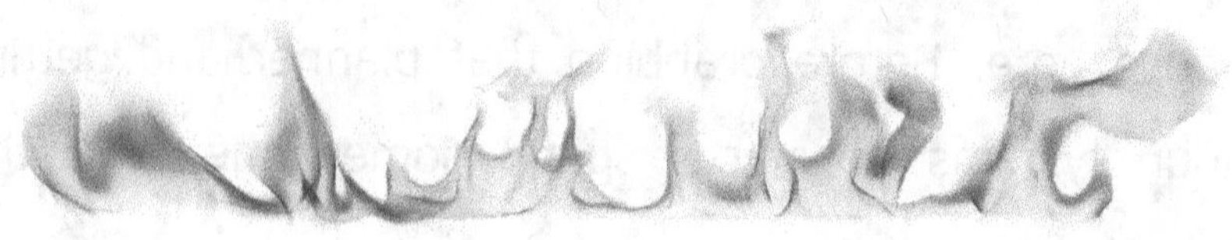

This chapter was added in the summer of 2020.
When the shit hit the fan.
As it sometimes does
When the crash comes
Or the call in the middle of the night
Or the Friday afternoon visit from the boss.
Fingertips weak, bleeding, raw
Let go
What they never held.
There is no going back.
What do we do now?
We go forward.

When the Crisis Comes:

Bouncing Forward

No amount of effort, prevention or consciousness can completely spare us the from cycles of loss which occur in life. If our internal fire is already flickering when devastation strikes, it is at risk of extinguishment. When darkness creeps in, the way forward becomes hard to see.

When you find yourself blindsided on your quest for the opposite of burnout, turn to this section. It provides an ordered plan to get you out of the darkness, to rekindle your fire so it can light your way.

The resources in this book will help you build a meaningful career. The references in this chapter will help you get back on your feet. Follow its seven steps, one after the other, to move from survival…to revival…to *THRIVAL*.

Resilience Defined

Resilience is not "bouncing back." Humans are forever changed by deep, disruptive experiences. True resilience involves release of the past, healing the losses and, eventually, embracing a new future. It takes time.

Resilience is not a gift you are either born with or not. It is a skillset you can gain, a process you can implement. Resilience is learned. Resilience is strengthened by practice, often over the course of an entire lifetime.

Human resilience is the ability to move forward from a crisis with a change in outlook, skills, expectations and capacity. By definition, to be resilient is to change. To be resilient is to be adaptable.

There are two types of Resilience. Type 1 (Primary) involves the capacity to:

- Change without having to experience a crisis,
- Change without accompanying trauma,
- Take action before it is forced.

Type 1 Resilience is *prevention*. Type 2 (Secondary) Resilience is *response*. It involves the capacity to:

- Recover after experiencing a crisis,
- Persist in the face of threat,
- Survive trauma and move forward.

Structured Resilience

Crisis dissipates energy and fractures focus. Suddenly, there is so much to take in, consider, respond to and deal with. Our limited energies are spent just trying to make sense of things, and we cannot get traction. Wheels spinning, we are depleted before we ever get off go.

Know the feeling?

Okay, pause. Take a breath. Imagine a stairwell before you, leading up and out, to a future you can't yet see. You're going to climb it, one step at a time, gaining strength and clarity as you rise, until you arrive at the top, energized and ready to move forward.

You can do this!

Follow the Seven Steps of Structured Resilience:

1. Triage
2. Rebuild Energy Reserves
3. Shift Your Sights - Long vision
4. Identify Needed Skills and Knowledge
5. Plan, But Differently
6. Implement with Ease
7. Prevention - Rebuild Capacity

These steps are strategically structured to move you up and out of crisis. To help you get your head on straight and regain traction toward your (perhaps new) dreams, just begin at the beginning. With whatever energy you can muster, focus on Step 1. Step 1 addresses the urgencies at hand while you regain some energy. Stay there until you notice your vitality and focus increase. It takes as long as it takes.

When you are ready, move to the next step, and the next and the next, regaining and compounding capacity at each level, and investing it in the next. Little by little you will get stronger, your light will get brighter, and you will find your way.

Step 1: Triage

Triage is a French word derived from the verb "trier," which means to choose, select, classify, sift, separate, and distinguish.

In the medical world, triage is an established process for determining life-saving priorities. Merriam-Webster defines **triage** as "the sorting of and allocation of treatment to patients and especially battle and disaster victims according to a system of priorities designed to maximize the number of survivors."

Triage is a systematic approach to quickly and effectively focus available resources toward the highest outcome.

Triage works:

> When chaos swirls…
> When we have limited focus or energy…
> When complications are coming at us fast and furiously…
> When the situation is constantly evolving…
> When the way is not clear…
> Now.

Any time you don't know where to begin, begin here, with triage. Use triage principles to pull your priorities out of the pile. Get a blank sheet of paper and get going on your first triage.

First, Get Clear

In order for triage to help you stay on track and protect life priorities, you have to know what those priorities are…at least in this moment. Begin each triage with the end in mind: on objective statement. We're not looking for a big Life Purpose here, just a way through the situation. Ask yourself:

- What do I want to experience today?
- What do I need most to show up as my best self so I can serve and support with my strengths?
- How do I want my life/work/relationship to look like when this crisis is over?
- What opportunity may be opening up for me to explore?
- What are my highest values?
- What do I need this triage to clarify for me?

Crystalize your confusion into a clear objective statement for this triage. Write it down on the top of your paper. Don't worry, you're not marrying it. You can change it for the next triage. The triage process only works if a clear outcome is defined.

Next, Dump

Spew everything onto the sheet of paper. Big, small, major, minor, work, personal—all of it. Get it out where you can see it. Keep going until you feel empty.

Pick Low-Hanging Fruit

Circle items which can be done quickly and free up energy, but don't relate to your priorities. On my list, low-hanging fruit might include housecleaning, quick administrative phone calls, online ordering, decluttering, and deleting emails. Since tasks like these can be energizing, save these for a time when your cognitive and/or physical energy are low. Set a timer or put on some energizing music and bang through these tasks.

Good Time to Get Help

Looking at these "low-hanging fruit" tasks ask yourself, who else could do these? If your initial response is, "No one," pin yourself down. Hold yourself to an answer. Challenge yourself to name names, whether they are employees, family members, friends or paid help. It's important to loosen your grasp on less important tasks so you can invest your limited energy in priorities. Consider this an exercise in letting go. The more you practice, the easier it gets.

Other questions to ask yourself at this point in the process:

- Can this task be automated or simplified?
- Can this task be eliminated, even if only temporarily?

- What support structures or systems could be put in place, involving other people, so the weight of these tasks is shared?
- What support can I give myself to reduce and/or manage my stress?

Once you've sifted out the dregs and are left with the big rocks, move to the next phase of triage.

Elevate YOUR Priorities

All tasks are NOT equal. Holding your objective statement in your heart, look over your list and put stars next to the 3 items which best support or align with it. Go fast here; don't think too hard. Because of the clearing you've done in the previous step, these top priorities may jump out and grab you. The energetic charge can be strong—don't ignore it. Honor it. Your intuition is wise.

Once you have 3 priorities—Only3! No exception!—now you must order them. Write "1" by the first priority, "2" by the second priority, and "3" by the third priority.

If your priorities do not come quickly, it means you need to recheck your objective statement and/or eliminate some low-hanging fruit. Try again.

Work It

Work your priorities in order, from the top down. Take breaks as needed, but stay on task. Start with Priority 1, complete it, and move to Priority 2. Stick with Priority 2 until it is done, and then move to Priority 3. When Priority 3 is done, so are you! Celebrate. Play. Rest. Restore. Hit the low-hanging fruit.

Let It Go

You got the important things done, so you're done! The remaining tasks don't matter. Those middle-level priority tasks have a special name: busy-work. Don't waste your energy on them. If, in a future triage, they rise to the top, you'll deal with them then.

Crumple up that sheet of paper and throw it away! Rest. Play. Restore.

And herein lies the beauty of triage. By getting clear on what is a priority, you also get clear on what isn't a priority. Letting go is an essential practice in stressful times, and triage helps you know what to let go of. Letting go is what will bring you peace. Letting go will give you space for the people, tasks and things to bring you joy. Let yourself fall into this new space you've created and receive the comfort and grounding it offers.

Repeat

Learn to recognize the need to triage. Whenever those feelings of overwhelm, confusion and anxiety begin to rise, pull out a blank sheet of paper and go through the process again, beginning with a fresh objective statement. The more you do it, the faster and easier it gets. Regular triage is a stress-busting habit which can serve you forever. TIP: Use the Habit Approach (discussed later) to retrain your brain to reach for triage instead of social media.

Step 2: Recover Energy

I know this about you: you are more exhausted than you realize. Whatever lead you to this chapter has depleted your energy. It was spent fighting to survive, prevent or recover from some unfortunate turn of events. You've drawn upon your reserves to mitigate damage or control outcomes.

And now you're here, on the edge of burnout.

While you keep the triage practice going, your next step toward resilience is to replenish your energy reserves. This step won't be hurried, so don't even try. It takes as long as it takes. Your willful mind can't hurry it. Your wise soul won't accept subterfuge. Your relationships can't be faked forever.

Consider how long it took you to slide into this low-energy state. Consider the collateral damage—to your body, emotions, mind, soul, relationships—needing time to heal. Factor in you are not only recovering energy, you are expending energy to deal with the current crisis, and you storing energy for the future.

Okay, you're probably starting to see this is a major effort requiring your full commitment. For life. Yes, resilience is a lifestyle. Take a moment to absorb this, to see yourself as a resilient person, to imagine a clear and energized you. This lies ahead for you. A journey of a thousand miles begins with the first step. Let this moment be that step.

From this moment, consider yourself MOVING IN THE DIRECTION OF greater and greater resilience. With this perspective, every experience provides support and direction for your journey. You're never off-course. You're always learning and growing toward greater resilience.

5 Forms of Energy

Your car probably has only one fuel tank, but you have five! They are separate but interconnected. The reserves of one can replenish another. Some are more readily accessed than others.

As you read about these 5 forms of energy, imagine a fuel gauge for each. What is your current level right now?

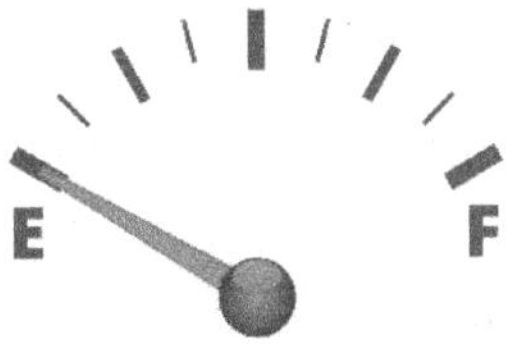

Physical energy: How strong does your body feel? What's your level of pep? Physical energy can be restored by sleep (EXTRA sleep in times of trauma or crisis!), nutrition, movement, daylight, and deep breathing. See Essential Strategy #1: Self Management for ways to increase physical energy.

Emotional energy: What's your level of positive feelings (hope, love, joy, gratitude, peace, etc)? Positive feelings can be generated by experiencing fun and inspiring moments; focusing on positive; decreasing internal and external stress; self-acceptance; adequate self-expression. See Non-Negotiable #5: Positive Mindset.

Cognitive energy: How clear is your thinking? How well can you sustain singular focus? To center your brain, challenge yourself to think creatively; reflect; focus and connect; decide and plan; learn to evolve and change. See Essential Strategy #5: Asset Protection.

Spiritual energy: Do you feel a connection to life purpose and meaning? What motivates you to keep going? Practices to increase spiritual energy include: mindfulness, meditation, walking in nature, journaling, religious practice, appreciative moments, connecting with nature, gratitude practice, developing faith, and learning about self as a spiritual being.

Relational and social energy: How strong are your connections with other people? Do you feel connected in a meaningful way with someone? As we go through life, meaningful connection takes attention and effort. Consciously build connection by being fully present with/for someone, connecting in conversation, or doing things together. You'll develop specific communication skills in Essential Strategy #4: Smart Communication.

Step 3. Lift Your Sights

In Step 1, you learned to triage. Triage is an orderly process for zeroing in on your priorities among the chaos surrounding you in any moment. Use Triage whenever confusion and overwhelm start to build. During times of crisis or burnout, triage is (at least) a daily practice. Triage will take care of the short term. Keep doing it.

In Step 2, you began the process of recovering your energy. This process takes as long as it takes and cannot be rushed. Attempting to rush it compromises your efforts and further depletes your precious reserves. Be patient. Keep resting and restoring all 5 types of energy.

You will know when it's time to move on to Step 3. Watch for these signs:

- A subtle, positive curiosity about what's ahead,
- Acceptance you're not going back to what was,
- Relief you're not going back to what was,
- A bubbling sense the future might, in some ways, be better than the past,
- An openness to possibilities.

Or, just ask yourself, "Am I ready to move forward?" When you sense, a "YES," go ahead and take the next step...

Look to the Future

In his book "Getting Things Done," David Allen presents what he calls Horizons of Focus. It's an airplane analogy, equating perspective with altitude. On the ground level runway, we focus on our instrument panel and the runway immediately before us. These represent the priorities at hand (triage). As we progressively gain altitude, our perspective shifts and broadens. We clear trees and buildings (projects). We follow landmarks and rivers (short-term goals and objectives). The horizon becomes more pronounced as we set our compass heading (long-term vision). Eventually, we clear the clouds (purpose and principles). Ideally, we periodically shift our Horizon of Focus as appropriate to monitor and maintain each perspective.

When you are in crisis, when chaos storms around you and your energy reserves are down, forget about all those horizons! Narrow your focus to just two levels: ground level and long-term vision.

Here's why…

Ground level priorities must be dealt with. If you don't practice regular triage, they'll scream until they get your attention. In this way, one way or another, ground level priorities *will* be handled.

Middle distance priorities—projects, goals and objectives—are in a state of flux. Trying to track on their everchanging state would consume inordinate amounts of your precious energy for very little return. You are unlikely to control them. Let them go for now.

Instead, set a compass heading and hold course for your future. Narrow your focus temporarily. What can you release, for now? At what level can you actively disengage from mid-level priorities? What outcomes can you release? What emotional investments can you withdraw? What might you completely stop giving energy to, for now? Be as specific as possible. Allow yourself to imagine crazy possibilities, after all, these are crazy times.

Finding Comfort in Your Long-Term Vision

Times of major change are perfect for long-term visioning.

When crisis or burnout has knocked you off your professional path, your long-term vision is a blank canvas. Isn't this intriguing? You can make your future whatever you want: a continuation of what you've known, a complete reboot, or anywhere in between. And there are some bonuses hidden here for you:

- You are so much wiser! You now know more about what you don't want to experience (whatever lead you to this dead end).
- You have more capacity going forward than ever! As a result of taking your time in Step 2, you now know more about what you need to sustain yourself.
- Nature is doing some of the hard work already! You are probably being forced to release some aspects of self and doing which were impeding your joyful path forward. You have the opportunity to grieve them, thank them, and let them go.

Move in the Direction of

A compass heading is enough for now. Keep your eyes on the 3-5 year horizon. Work to gain clarity of what you want to experience more of in your life. If anything were possible (and it is!), what would your perfect life look and feel like in 3-5 years? Allow yourself to dream. Write down key words. Involve your loved ones who will share this future.

Imagine enjoying and sustaining high levels of all forms of personal energy: physical, emotional, cognitive, spiritual, relational and social.

Consider all areas of your life: career, money, health, friends and family, significant other/romance, personal growth, fun and recreation, home, spiritual connection.

As you form this vision of your future, you are activating the "Moving in the Direction of" principle. Your action is rewarded. You receive clarity and guidance. You understand more. Resources and support appear. Interferences fall away.

Putting positive energy into what you want to experience in the future creates an energetic field which pulls you toward it. Setting your intention for what you want to experience programs your brain to identify the quickest route to achieving it. Focusing on what feels good leverages your positive neurotransmitters and activates the Upward Spiral.

For a more structured approach to developing your long-term vision, see Essential Strategy #2: Personal Branding. Exercises include:

> SWOT Analysis
> List Mining
> Life Review
> Jack Canfields Mission Statement Exercise
> Consult the Experts

The Bounce Begins

Stay with this step—Developing a Long-Term Vision—until you sense a shift. Maybe you'll notice something beginning to solidify. Like a crystallization from the fog. Or your future beginning to color in. Do you feel it?

This is the other gift of a structured resilience process: after you've triaged, and recovered some energy, and invested it in developing a vision of your future, something clicks in. It can be subtle, but it will come. Look for it. Gears engaging. Initial traction. Forward pull. Maybe even hope. This is your signal you are ready to move to Step 4.

Step 4: Identify Needed Skills and Knowledge

If your journey were depicted in a graphic novel, our hero would be standing at the precipice of a giant canyon with a big question mark overhead. How do we get from where we've been to where we want to go? For many professionals, the first step is a doozy! It requires faith you can take a step and a bridge will appear.

Restoring Faith

Of course your faith is shaken. How could it not be when the unimaginable has caught you by surprise. Remind yourself:

- You've built your life and career before, so you can do it again.
- You've got to be somewhere in 5 years (choose any period in the future), so you might as well determine where that will be.
- You offer something special and unique someone needs and is willing to pay you for.
- Times change, so adaptation is a skill you need in order to survive and thrive. You are developing this skill now.
- Seizing this opportunity to build a positive future is the best way to insure one.
- Your past achievements and successes prove you've got what it takes.

The reason mindset is a "non-negotiable" (see Non-Negotiable #5: Positive Mindset) is you've already got one. The default mindset is negative. To support our survival, your primitive brain was programmed to look for danger/bad/negative. It takes consciousness and commitment—beginning with a decision!—to reprogram your brain for positivity.

Now is the time to decide to commit to a positive future.

Embracing the Unknowing

For many professionals, sense of self is built upon what we know. Knowing/learning is where we invested many years and many dollars. Knowing/learning is what we offer our clients. What we know is our image, our cache, our differentiator.

When we're so vested in our knowing, it's very hard to step into unknowing, but that's what is needed now. You see, you've reached the limits of your knowing. At this point, your knowing is probably getting in your way.

Consider the Four Stages of Knowing:

1. You don't know what you don't know (Unconscious Incompetence)
2. You know what you don't know (Conscious Incompetence)
3. You know what you know (Conscious Competence)
4. You don't know what you know (Unconscious Competence)

As a professional, you've probably reached Stage 4, Unconscious Competence. It is that effortless, riding-a-bike level of expertise which makes you good at your work. The problem with Stage 4 is there is nowhere to go from there. You're all filled up. There's no room to learn. Continuing to clutch what you know makes you blind to what you need to know.

It's time to find the humility and curiosity of a child and face Stage 1, wondering what you don't know. This is where things get interesting. And exciting!

Exploring the Gap

Hey you, our Hero, standing at that precipice…

Behind you is a long and winding path which led you here. It has served you well but it can take you no farther. On the other side you see your future, a 3-5 year vision that's becoming clearer and clearer. Let's explore what it will take to get you from here to there. Get rooted in that place of curious unknowing. Playfully explore these routes of discovery:

- **Skills inventory** - Discover which of your skills can transfer to unforeseen positions, as well as the skills you'll need to acquire. A broad (cross-industry) Skills Inventory exercise can reveal both (see resource page at https://LizGarrett.com/opposite/).
- Interviews - Conduct broad internet searches for people who are already doing the work you'd like to do. Ask to interview them. Have a prepared list of questions and listen deeply to their responses. Show humility and gratitude. As scary as this may be, it is so worthwhile. You have NOTHING to lose and so much to gain, including a powerful ally. Do it.
- Get coached - A certified professional coach is specifically trained to draw out your best strengths in support of your goals. Because they keep you focused and moving forward, the time-savings and clarity they facilitate is a worthwhile investment.
- Research job ads for your dream job - Not that you're going to apply (but you can!), reading job ads for dream positions tells you specifically what qualities or qualifications you need to be able to show on your resume.

This due diligence will result in a list of skills you need to develop. Move on to Step 5, Plan, But Differently

Step 5: Plan, But Differently

I know you know how to plan, so let's not even go there.

You know planning is important. Planning is a map to the future you desire. Planning helps you accomplish, step by step, your dream. Planning is good, so plan. But....

Planning also contributed to the mess you're in. Planning blinded you to important signs.

Your Brain's Secrets

I'm going to let you in on some secrets your brain is keeping from you.

Your brain does not always have your best interest in mind.

You know what else? Your brain thinks it's the boss of you. Yep. Isn't that funny?

And the last thing—and this is the worst—your brain has no heart. Nope. It would like you to believe it can *think* its way into feeling. But thoughts are not feelings. Feelings are the domain of the heart, and for many of us, heart and brain are not on speaking terms.

In case your brain is listening and starting to get upset, let me be clear: Brain, we love you! Our powerful human brain is capable of so much. Brain, no one is doubting your awesomeness!

But brain alone CANNOT lead you to happiness, true success, or your highest potential. For that, you're going to need to harness and direct all of who you are: mind, body and spirit; inner/outer; past, present and future.

Are you ready to enjoy greater creativity and productivity? Engage in meaningful work? Appreciate deeper relationships? Laugh more. Hurt less. Enjoy better sleep? Less stress and anxiety?

You're going to have to sort of trick your powerful brain into working _for_, not against, you.

(Shhhhhh) Brain doesn't even have to know it.

Planning vs Unplanning

This is tricky, this balance. I'm speaking from experience. I am someone who once delighted in goal maps, and planners, and progress charts, and monthly checkpoints. Someone who wrote a 24-page workbook for goal setting (available for free download at https://LizGarrett.com/opposite/). Someone who is a professional coach.

I've always been goal-oriented. At the beginning of each year, I was deep in markers and highlighters and planners and spreadsheets, laying out a detailed and color-coded map for where I want to go in the year ahead.

And then, a review of my planner/journals revealed:

- **Willfulness accomplishes very little.** For the effort and time I put into pages and pages of planning, I got very little direct return. More of my plans didn't go as planned as did, and those which did work out would have worked out without my planning. Yet, my over-arching goals, including financial, were met or exceeded.
- **The focus on the destination diminishes the journey.** The necessary tunnel vision of goal-orientation activates a harsh self-discipline which spawns guilt or perceived failure or, at the very least, a slight shutting down to unexpected pleasures which present themselves in the moment. I've come to believe those unexpected

pleasures are important expressions of our heart, and should be explored.

- **(Metaphoric) Mid-winter is the wrong time of year to plant seeds.** Nature is sleeping, and we are part of nature. Winter is a time to go slow or even stop. It's time to sleep and dream. It's time to synthesize, to integrate. It is a waste of energy to fight Nature; she always wins. Slow down with Nature's slow-down. Things get so much easier when we honor the cycles of Nature planted within us.

I bet you can relate.

The Problem with Goals

If this heresy offends you, I understand. Ten years ago I tried to read a book called "Goal-Free Living." I was so appalled by its concepts, I didn't finish it. It was like a slap in the face, so counter to the goal-oriented principles I was deeply committed to at the time. Recently I dug it out of the depths of my Kindle library for a revisit. It makes more sense now. The author, Stephen M. Shapiro, offers these Eight Secrets of Goal-Free Living:

1. Use a compass, not a map.
2. Trust you are never lost.
3. Remember opportunity knocks often, but sometimes softly.
4. Want what you have.
5. Seek out adventure.
6. Become a people magnet.
7. Embrace your limits.
8. Remain detached.

Goals are a given. We are all responsible professionals committed to meeting certain business outcomes. We have to meet our metrics. We have to pay our bills. But, really? Isn't that a low bar? Goals are our payment to Caesar. Goals are the price of admission. Goals are the wand, not the wizard. A joyful, lucrative, sustainable career (life!) has got to be about more than goals!!! To engage in an artful dance of intention and attention, to find meaning in the mundane, to home in on our heart's desire in the service of others…now, this, THIS MAKES IT WORTH THE EFFORT.

What We Can't Un-Know Now

Deriving large parts of my professional identity as someone who maps out goals and achieves them gave me a smug self-confidence, a sense of security I could "make" things happen. Ha!

Let me ask you, what were your plans for the year in January 2020?

> *"Life is what happens to you while you're busy making other plans." -John Lennon*

Goal-focus lost its magic for me. The mojo is gone. It suddenly looks to me like a lot of hubris. Energy wasted. Focus on the future at the expense of the present, where there are beautiful sunsets and roses every day. Focusing on the future gave me a FALSE confidence and sense of security. Focus on the future kept me limited by my abilities and resources, blind to unseen forces which rally on my behalf.

And that's the point. Finding the strength to keep my focus in the present—despite the pressure to pull it forward into the future—accesses *GREATER* resources, guidance and power. Right here, right now. That's where everything happens. Nothing happens in the future.

In the Absence of Goals

Reducing goals to a minor, subsistence role in your life frees a lot of space. For now, do your best to keep this space empty. To simply hold it. Holding space…isn't that a cool mental image? Keeping the space empty for something. For what? For knowing. For joy. Love. The Unexpected.

Holding Space is a coaching principle. I like the simple way Michael Bungay Stanier describes it in "*The Coaching Habit:*" Don't rush to action. Stay curious.

Usually "holding space" implies holding space for another person. What if we gave this gift to ourselves?

Where the Real Work Is

Holding space is active, not passive, and it's harder than it sounds. The pull forward is strong. The inner critic is loud. The fear monster manically points toward a future you "should" be controlling. As if you could. Ha.

Think of a garden: a neat rectangle cut into the earth to hold space for the tomatoes and zucchini and cantaloupe. We certainly have a role—prepare the soil, plant the seeds, tend the growth—but the garden grows on its own.

Your job, right now, is to prepare the soil, plant the seeds and tend the growth. Be curious about what's growing in your garden. Watch for sprouts. Pull weeds. Choose, over and over, a thousand times over, to trust Nature's process.

Whole-Brain Planning

Let this point in your rebuilding be a pivot point, an opportunity to forever change your approach to planning. Learn to plan loosely, in a balanced way. Be alert to your left brain's desire to jump back into its seat of control and command. Remember, your left brain, unchecked, got you into this mess.

The brain's two hemispheres have different functions. To leverage our full potential, we want to access both hemispheres in a balanced way. If your work has drawn upon your left-brain capacities, now is an excellent time to lean into right-brain dominance. Begin to approach planning in a way which involves BOTH sides of your brain. It will feel different for you, maybe a little scary, so give yourself time to find your way with this.

Left Brain Functions	**Right Brain Functions**
• Decisions	• Emotions
• Logic	• Intuition
• Thinking in words	• Creativity
• Numbers	• Visualization
• Critical Thinking	• Rhythm
• Reasoning	• Imagination
• Facts	• Art

Balanced-brain planning looks like this:

- Ebb and flow; dance-like; yin and yang; inward and outward focus,
- Left brain identifies *what* needs to be done; right brain decides *when* and *how,*
- Flowy, subject to change,
- Gentle, kind, self-accepting,
- If things don't get done, it's okay, because key insights and information are gleaned,
- Heart is heard and engaged in process,
- All 5 energy levels are monitored and supported,

- Guided by bigger Vision,
- More joy, deeper satisfaction, greater ease.

Shift your approach to planning by committing to key practices supporting Whole-Brain engagement. Make them habitual. Build them into your day. Put them on your calendar. Set expectations with loved ones and colleagues. You'll have to figure out what works for you—which will change—but here's a good starting place:

- Regular self-reflection supported by objective feedback and personal measures
- Periods of stillness, recovery, restoration
- Morning Margins – to check in with self, set tone for day
- Evening Margins – to review and appreciate day

The "One Perfect Day" workbook (download free at https://LizGarrett.com/opposite/) leads you through the Integrated Journaling™ process combining journaling and planning for all-day, everyday consciousness. **Journaling + Planning = Focus**. Focus is on a specific goal, but the goal can change. Personalized measures are used to provide somewhat objective feedback and direction. It is important to adapt Integrated Journaling to your existing organizational style, and this workbook will show you how.

So, go ahead, plan. Plan joyfully. Plan playfully. Plan with curious expectancy. Plan with a loose grip.

Enter the dance.

Step 6: Implement with Ease

It's okay for things to be occasionally *challenging*. Challenges make you stronger. Challenges increase capacity. Challenges have the quality of moving WITH the flow. Challenges lead you in the direction of your dreams.

In contrast, *struggle* is a red flag. Struggle has the quality of AGAINST. Struggle is a battle. Struggle is uphill. Struggle depletes. Struggle is trying to tell you something. Possibly:

- Ego has taken over and is "willing" at your expense.
- You need to make a change.
- You need more support.
- You're out of balance, out of the flow, out of joy.
- It's time to coarse correct.

As you move forward with your plan, seek ease. Ease tells you you are in the flow. Ease provides guidance and resources when you need them. Ease uplifts and carries. Ease is, well, easy.

The struggle/ease dichotomy is one of the easiest direction indicators to learn and use. Pay attention to what feels like struggle and what feels like ease. At every fork in the road, choose ease over struggle and watch the joyful, meaningful path unfold before you.

Enlist your brain as your ally in ease. By leveraging two processes your brain is already doing—intention and habits—you direct your brain's massive resources to work for—not against—you.

Leverage Intention

Your mind is always going to be doing something, why not have it work in auto-pilot for your benefit? Setting empowering intentions is as simple as deciding what you want to experience in a situation. It can be done at any time for any situation: at the beginning of each day; at any point within any relationship; to manifest a particular project outcome; to affect health conditions; to redirect financial circumstances; to experience pleasant travel; to support specific goals; and, at any point you want to turn around a negative experience. Here are some guidelines for developing empowering intentions:

1. **Empowering Intentions are based in reality.** Intention must relate to the challenge as well as the goal. Intention is not wishing.

2. **Empowering Intentions acknowledge feelings.** Feelings are your friend. They carry a lot of energy, and this energy attracts the object of those feelings. The more you infuse intentions with positive words and meanings which matter to you, the more powerful they will be.

3. **Empowering Intentions focus on moving toward, not away from.** State intentions in terms of what you are manifesting. Avoid the word "not."

4. **Empowering Intentions are stated in the present tense.** State your intention as if it has already come true. Think of it as an existing reality which you are now choosing to join.

5. **Empowering Intentions are in alignment with Universal forces.** There are forces greater than you, natural laws which you will not change. Seek to observe and understand these so your intentions are powered by their flow.

6. **Empowering Intentions require you to claim what is possible for your life.** Sometimes the hardest thing about building a good, happy, productive, fulfilling life is deciding what it will look like… and then actively claiming it.

(Excerpt from *Intentionology: 365 Days of Living on Purpose* by Liz Garrett)

Leverage Habits

Your behavior is driven by habits. Already today, you have operated dozens (or more) times in autopilot. Your behaviors, including your emotional responses, are driven by cue, routine, reward – the Habit Loop described by Charles Duhigg in <u>The Power of Habit</u>.

The question is, are your habits working FOR or AGAINST you?

Life gets easier when you take advantage of your brain's autopilot feature. Habits are powerful, but delicate. They will operate in perfect mechanized precision until you intentionally change the program.

Duhigg tells us our brains operate in a habit loop. A **cue** stimulates the brain to drive a thought or behavior (**routine**) to create the **reward** it seeks.

Once you know how, reprogramming your habits is one of the easiest—and most powerful!—things you can do to begin to redirect your life. Here's how…

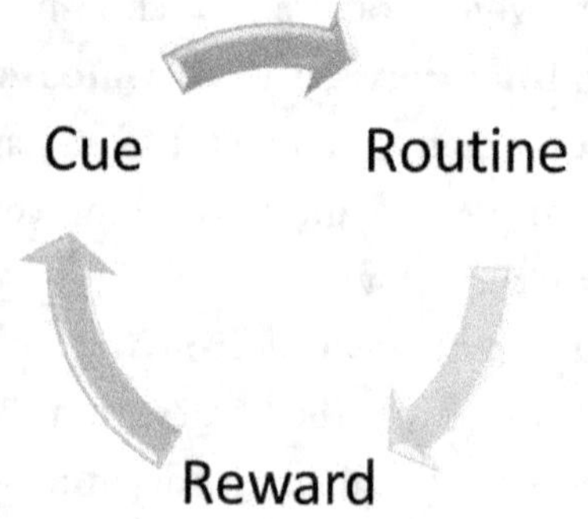

Change Your Habits in 3 Easy Steps:

1. **Observe cues**. Cues trigger behavior, consciously or unconsciously. Cues may include thoughts, images, times of day, visual triggers, places, emotions, company of certain people. Cues might be as solid as your feet hitting the floor in the morning, or as ephemeral

as the fear of being judged. Cues turn on your habit loop. Knowing—or creating—your cues is how you will leverage the habit loop.

2. **Observe your rewards**. What are the payoffs you crave? Rewards may be *physical*, like certain sensations, foods or experiences. Often the rewards we crave are *emotional*, such as the feelings of love and belonging, or justification for anger and loneliness. Understand what drives your habits. You're not going to deny your rewards; you're going to find healthier ways to create them.

3. **Change your routines**. Between cue and reward, insert a different behavior. This can be as simple or complex as you want. For example, if you want to experience increased strength and energy (reward), start the habit of putting on running shoes (routine) as soon as your feet hit the floor (cue). If you want to experience greater closeness in your relationship (reward), start the habit of asking your partner about their day (routine), when they walk through the door each evening (cue). These are just examples. To see how I used these principles to shift my wake-up habit, read Teaching an Old Brain New Tricks and download The Lazy Brain Goal-Sheet (https://LizGarrett.com/blog).

It really is this easy: identify the outcome you seek, and hang a new habit on an existing cue. Once the habit becomes ingrained, it will become the brain's new autopilot, and you will experience the results you desire, effortlessly! Little by little, habit by habit, you are moving in the direction of your dreams.

Step 7: Prevention - Rebuild Capacity

Dawn is breaking on a new day for you. Rays of light slice through parting clouds. Pure potential abounds. A new journey begins. You are ready to step forward.

With each step of resilience recovery, you built momentum which carried you to the next step, which built momentum for the next, and so on, lifting you upward toward greater strength and focus. Look how far you've come! Continue the Upward Spiral. Strategically leverage the powerful forces you've set into motion to establish practices which prioritize your well-being. Fiercely monitor and protect your five types of energy: Physical, Emotional, Cognitive, Spiritual, and Relational/Social.

Here are 3 specific things to do RIGHT NOW, sweet opportunities available at this critical juncture.

#1 Create a Resilience Journal

Take advantage of this upswing to gain awareness and create a record of what lifts/supports/sustains you. YOU! This is a special space in time to unlock YOUR secret resilience combination. Designate a small notebook, or Bullet Journal pages, or space in your planner for your Resilience Journal:

- 20 - 30 pages should be enough.
- Put headings at the top of each page.
  - Example headings can be downloaded from Crisis Resources (https://LizGarrett.com/opposite/).
  - Make them meaningful to you by adding or deleting headings.
- Carry the notebook with you and make lists under each heading.
- You are writing notes to your future self, a breadcrumb trail out of challenging times.
- Reference your notes when you notice your energy levels declining.

#2 Renegotiate Expectations

This is your ebb tide moment. Forces greater than you are creating change. Don't fight the tide. Ride it!

Maybe there are some things/relationships/efforts/projects you want to let go.

Maybe there are some things/relationships/efforts/projects you want to begin.

Maybe there are some things/relationships/efforts/projects you want to change.

Now is your chance!

Consider your obligations to spouse, children, parents, employers, community, neighbors, volunteer activities, even pets. Which ones bring you joy, and which do not? Which restore your energy, and which do not? If you ever wanted to make a change, the tide is now on your side.

Here are some renegotiation conversation starters:

- "I want to talk about the way we [do this thing], and make some changes which work for both of us."
- "[X] used to work for me, but it doesn't anymore. Here is what I'm doing going forward…and here is what I need from you."
- "A lot is changing for me right now, so I am letting some things go, including [x]. Here is what you can expect from me in the phase-out."
- Start sentences with "I" as much as possible. Notice what comes up when you use "I" statements. This is pure gold.
- It's okay to say, "Yesterday I felt that way and today I feel this way," if that's your truth.
- "It's important I begin [x]. Here is what I need from you to support me. What can you commit to?"
- "I'm making some changes to create a future I can get excited about. Here is what I'd like to see for us…"

Be compassionate and allow the recipient some time to process this information. Be prepared to use the "broken record" technique, repeating the same message verbatim several times before they actually hear it. You will find more guidelines in Essential Strategy #4: Smart Communication.

#3 Double-Down on Pleasure

Your body is wired to associate pleasure with its five sensory inputs: sight, sound, touch, taste and smell. When change is occurring all around you, grounding into your physical body is very stabilizing. Observing what brings you pleasure initiates the Upward Spiral, assuring you'll experience more and more pleasure. Pleasure points you down a joyful path. Pleasure is your breadcrumb trail to your internal flame. Learn to follow it.

The easiest—and most delightful—thing you'll do all day is simply tune into your senses! It requires no money, no time, no equipment, no assistance, nor another person. Yet, it will allow you to fall more fully into yourself, to be present to the beauty of your mere existence. Try it now:

- Lift your eyes from this page and let them survey your surroundings. Feel as they drink in your favorite colors, flit across meaningful objects, and soak in the comforts surrounding you. See rays of light which left the Sun only eight minutes ago dance on the surfaces around you, only to be received by your eyes.
- Now, close your eyes and let your ears "see" for you. Go past the identification and labeling of the sounds—cat purring, train passing, distant wind chimes—and simply take in life's symphonic vibration.
- Lightly run your fingers along your body. Feel the nerve endings in your sensitive hands come alive as they process the voluptuous textures of your clothing, the warmth of your skin, the silkiness of

your hair. Did you also feel yourself exhale and relax to your own touch?

- When you put food in your month, notice the playground on your tongue! Your taste buds discern salty, sweet, sour, bitter and umami (savory), and your brain converts the signals into pure primal pleasure! Fully give in to the "mmmmmmm" of your next meal.

- Smell, the most powerful of all your senses, is the only one going straight to your emotional brain, making you feel before you can think. Without your awareness, you are constantly processing as many as 10,000 scents which directly influence not only your emotions, but also most of your body's major systems. Use this to make yourself feel good! Breathe in soothing frankincense, grounding ginger, uplifting lemon, or sexy ylang ylang to immediately feel what you want to feel.

Create "The Opposite of Burnout" Lifestyle

The remaining chapters present burnout prevention as a lifestyle. You will find actionable practices you can adopt, strategies to implement, to support you in building and sustaining your energy reserves.

Essential Strategy #1: Self-Management

Your body is your vehicle for life. You will only go as far as it takes you. Just like your car requires basic care and maintenance, your body is a machine with certain requirements in order to function. For optimal, sustainable functioning—for you to be and do all you want to be and do in this life—your body's basic needs must be met. Learn simple strategies for accommodating the 5 Non-Negotiables and the sanity-saving practice of "Moving in the Direction Of."

Tools Provided In This Chapter: 10% More, Reference List – Foods You Like, Lifestyle Strategies For Better Nutrition, Sleep Commitment Exercise, Better Sleep Habits, Better Sleep Plan, More Activity Plan, Stress Red Flags Check-Off, Stress-Prep Chart, Tools And Reminders To Beat Stress, 100% Responsibility Exercise, Difficult Or Troubling Situation Exercise.

Essential Strategy #2: Personal Branding

Personal branding is about presenting yourself to others to engage them in what you want to accomplish: your mission. Personal Branding is consciously developed from within. Personal Branding is a valuable counter to burnout because it enables you to release the trivial b.s. which creates stress and subterfuge, while keeping you focused on what matters…to YOU.

Tools Provided In This Chapter: SWOT Analysis, 3 Tools For Finding Your Mission Statement, Brand Action Plan, Reflection, Upward Spiral

Essential Strategy #3: Mindful Organization

When insides don't match outsides, there is friction. Think of that friction as fueling the fire of burnout. Let's reduce the friction by making sure the way you use your space, time and actions reflects your best self and highest potential. *Mindful* organization goes beyond arbitrary neatness and efficiency. *Mindful* organization consciously leverages your space, time and tasks to launch you toward your idea of success with greater ease and joy. *Mindful* organization is strategic and purposeful, and very, very personal. Live your life according to your terms and priorities so you can enjoy a long, fruitful career by developing and maintaining mindfulness in three pervasive dimensions: Space, Time and Tasks.

Tools Provided In This Chapter: "Busy" Awareness, Tips For Mindful Organization With Microsoft Outlook, "Multitasking" Awareness, "Time

States" Awareness, Agenda For Room Function Discussion, Clutter Awareness, Task Tips.

Essential Strategy #4: Smart Communication

Communication skills are your #1 promotability factor, more important than your education, experience, popularity, ambition or tenacity. Set yourself apart with smart communication skills that:

- Build alliances,
- Focus on specific desired outcomes,
- Strategize at least 3 steps out,
- Give up "Being Right" in favor of "Being Effective,"
- Get you more of what you want so you beat burnout.

Tools Provided In This Chapter*: Communication Skills Self-Assessment, Social Predictor Test, Guidelines For Authentic Communication, Strategies For Breaking Dynamic Tension, How To Adjust Communication For DISC, Guidelines For Communicating Leadership, Formula For Saying "No," S.P.I.R.A.L.*

Essential Strategy #5: Asset Protection

Your brain is your greatest professional asset. Its speed and capacity far exceeds any computer. Unlike a computer, a healthy brain has the awesome ability to create new neural pathways and alter existing ones to accommodate learning, processing experiences, and forming memories, for your entire life. Learn the care and feeding of your brain, as well as how to undo damage and create new circuitry so you can beat burnout.

Tools Provided In This Chapter*: 5 Ways To Care For Your Brain, 8 Practices For Creating New Circuitry.*

A Potentially Unpopular P.S.

There's something else needing to be said.

During the pandemic crisis, we saw instances where resilience was twisted and used as a weapon against others in three ways: Shaming, Shoulding and Misappropriation. These three forms of resilience abuse are related and interconnected.

This was evident as employees shifted quickly to working from home. Mostly without missing a beat, they set up home work-spaces, communications, and technology. Concurrently, many experienced additional stresses as their loved ones struggled with change and potential illness. At a time when the five types of personal energy needed to be restored and preserved, it was tapped to continue the mission of their work. When they experienced weariness or unclear thinking, they wondered what was wrong with them. When deadlines loomed, they quietly worked into the nights and weekends. Few had conversations about revising expectations under the circumstances. Workers felt they "should" be able to handle this. They suffered in silence to avoid shame and judgement. Employers saw results and didn't hit the pause button to redefine the mission, regroup around needs, and reassign resources.

Here's the thing…Any of us could be guilty of any of these, especially during time of crisis. When our resilience starts to wane and our fears kick in, we can unconsciously become part of someone else's problem.

Take a moment, take a breath, and take a humble look inside for any of these signs:

Resilience Shaming

Often an offshoot of various forms of privilege, Resilience Shaming assumes everyone should be able to cope as well as you do.

Examples of Resilience Shaming:

- Any form of comparison which implies an individual's resilience is inadequate.
- Negatively judging an individual for how they deal with crisis.
- Implying fault.

Correction:

- Tap into your compassion. It is impossible to know the circumstances of another's suffering.
- Create safe space for a person to express their needs. Listen to understand.
- If they request specific assistance, provide it if you can.

Resilience Shoulding

Thinking you know what others need to do to build their resilience is about you, your comfort level, and how they fit into your needs; it's not about them. You can't possibly know the path of their soul's growth.

Examples of Resilience Shoulding:

- Trying to "fix" another person.
- Implementing broad-brush resilience programs in the workplace.
- Prescribing one-size-fits-all resilience formula.

Correction:

- Focus on your own resilience, since "Shoulding" may be a projection of your own needs onto others.
- Work to understand the resilience needs of people you care about, in *their* terms.

Resilience Misappropriation

Resilience belongs solely to the individual. An employer, spouse or family member has no right to draw upon any individual's resilience. Resilience cannot be required or expected of an individual to justify mistreatment, abuse or neglect.

Examples of Resilience Appropriation:

- Not providing an employee with adequate resources to create the desired outcome, while expecting the employee to draw upon their resilience to get the job done.
- Not respecting an individual's stated needs, yet expecting them to meet yours.

Correction:

- Provide for their needs; support their resilience.
- Adjust expectations about outcomes.
- Increase your own capacity to reduce your requirements of others.

◆◆◆

Let this chapter be a resource and refuge for tough times. Come back to it any time you feel stuck or challenged so you can regain clarity and forward motion. At the same time, allow the following 5 Essential Strategies to form an ever-evolving framework for your success and satisfaction.

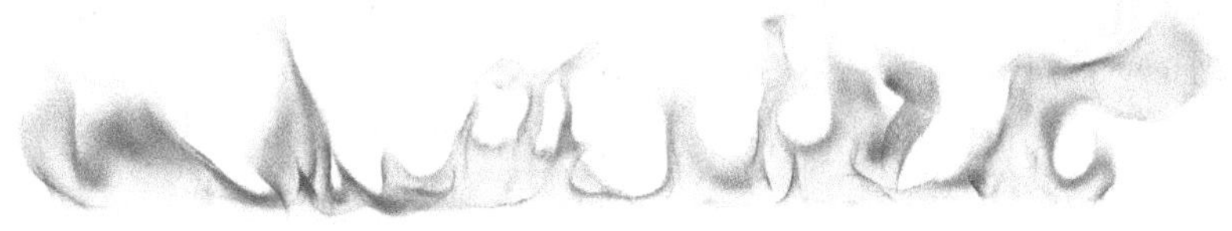

Essential Strategy #1:

Self-Management

YOUR BODY IS YOUR VEHICLE for life. You will only go as far as it takes you. Just like your car requires basic care and maintenance, your body is a machine that has certain requirements in order to function. Unlike your car, however, your body is highly complex and has contingency systems built in that allow you to go for some time, for example, without proper fuel (nutrition). Contingency systems operate at greater expense. These contingency systems fool you into thinking you can disregard your body's requirements forever. You cannot.

For optimal, sustainable functioning—for you to be and do all you want to be and do in this life—your body's basic needs must be met. It has 5 Non-Negotiables: nutrition, sleep, activity, stress management, and mindset. If you think you can justify compromising them, you're fooling yourself. If you think you are beating them, you're losing. That's why they are NON-NEGOTIABLE.

No need to make this difficult. No need to psychoanalyze your issues. No need to "should" all over yourself. Just "move in the direction" of increased self-management.

Moving in the Direction Of

This is a low-stress, high-results approach to achieving your goals. In each choice, just try to move a little closer to your desired outcome than you are now. That's all. Make this approach a way of life and you will see yourself move steadily toward your dreams.

> ## Jack Canfield asks,
> ## "What will it take to do just 10% more?"

The 5 Non-Negotiables

Non-Negotiable #1: Nutrition

Earning my Biology degree, one of the toughest classes I took was Cell Biology, and the most feared exam question was this: Describe the Krebs Cycle. As you can see, it is a highly complex, highly precise series of chemical reactions that occurs in each of the 100 trillion cells in your body. This sequence is how the body produces energy, one cell at a time. There are many more similar sequences going on, all the time, for other important functions.

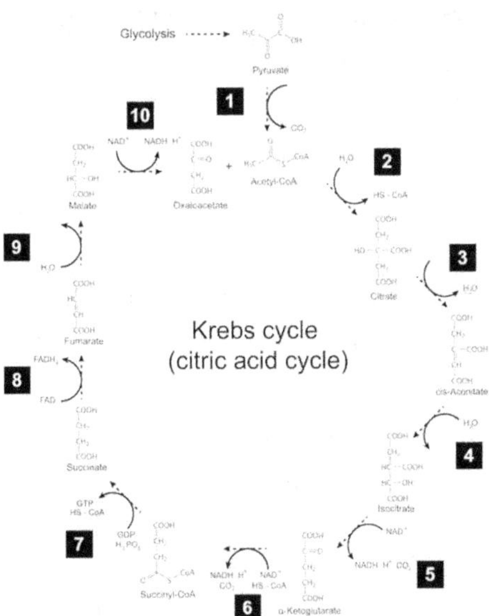

I passed the class, the test and, I suppose, that exam question, but I can no longer spout out the various reactions and equations that are occurring.

What did get deeply embedded in my understanding is this: cells require certain carbohydrates, fats and proteins to function properly. The systems are complex enough that there are some "emergency bypass routes" available to the cells if they don't have everything they need. But those are for short-term use only. If deprived of the nutrients they need and forced to use these emergency bypass routes long-term, failure occurs. What is failure? At first it is less-than-optimal function, and then it is disease, and then it is death.

Your Body's Minimum Fuel Requirements:

Putting nutritionally void foods in your body is like putting sand in your car's tank. Don't expect to go far. Your body needs:

- A variety of vegetables from all of the subgroups—dark green, red and orange, legumes (beans and peas), starchy, and other
- Fruits, especially whole fruits
- Grains, at least half of which are whole grains
- Fat-free or low-fat dairy, including milk, yogurt, cheese (or no dairy)
- A variety of protein foods, including seafood, lean meats and poultry, eggs, legumes (beans and peas), and nuts, seeds, and soy products
- Healthy Oils (olive, coconut, nut oils)
- Limited or no Saturated fats and *trans* fats, added sugars, and sodium

> ## 🗎 Develop a reference list of the foods you like in each category.
>
> Keep this list in your system for easy reference.

How can you MOVE IN THE DIRECTION OF better nutrition?

You do not need to become a nutritional expert, nor do you need to forgo food you enjoy. Deprivation doesn't work. Life—and food—are meant to be enjoyed. A little bit of anything won't hurt you. These two simple strategies will help:

1. Plan better.
2. Choose closer to earth.

Strategy One: Plan Better

Powerful commercial interests work against your healthy choices. There is money to be made selling nutritionally sparse food you, literally, can't get enough of. Well-funded, sophisticated marketing campaigns constantly influence your choices. It takes effort and awareness to eat well, but it's easier than you think. ✓ Check-off planning strategies you want to try:

- ☐ Create a file of good recipes you enjoy making and eating. Keep the ingredients on hand.
- ☐ Double, or even, triple recipes so you have leftovers to eat the next day or freeze for the future.
- ☐ Take advantage of your grocery store's online shopping service. It memorizes your list so that you can check-off items in a matter of minutes, and drive by for your groceries on your way home from work.
- ☐ Stock your kitchen and office with healthy snacks you will grab when you're hungry. Remove junk food from your reach.
- ☐ Do your research once and make lists you can reference when you're hungry and hurried. Lists like: Healthy Fast Food Choices, Healthy Restaurant Food, Snacks I Enjoy, Dessert Options, etc.
- ☐ Subscribe to an online meal delivery service for some or all of your meals.
- ☐ Schedule meal-planning and preparation into your week. This could be a family event.

Strategy Two: Choose Close to the Earth

Choosing healthy food should not be stressful! Just do your best in the moment to "move in the direction of" better nutrition by selecting the option that is closer to its natural form. Follow the food chain and choose the item closest to the sun. Survey what's available and select the food that is closest to its natural whole form. Look for ingredients you recognize; no chemicals or additives. It's a lifestyle, not a diet. Check-off strategies you might try:

- ☐ In a convenience store, choose vacuum-packed carrots and hummus rather than chips.

- ☐ At a restaurant, choose grilled or broiled chicken rather than breaded, fried chicken with gravy.
- ☐ At a buffet, fill your plate with salad, vegetables and lean protein.
- ☐ When hosted for dinner, take larger portions of salad, vegetables and lean protein, and smaller portions of bread, cream dishes, starches, and desserts.
- ☐ For breakfast on-the-go, grab a boiled egg rather than a power bar.
- ☐ When you have a choice of bread, choose whole grain.
- ☐ Choose foods with ingredients you recognize and can pronounce.
- ☐ Opt for whole foods, not processed foods.

Non-Negotiable #2: Sleep

I know, I know. There are so many more important things to do than sleep. Maybe, at some level, you pride yourself on how little you sleep, mentioning it to people like a badge of honor. A guy I once worked with, "Daniel," bragged that he only needed 5 hours of sleep; "that's just how he was wired." Daniel also couldn't write on a sticky note without first penciling perfectly horizontal guidelines using a ruler. He exhibited OCD-level control over everything his department produced, but he, himself, produced very little. Yeah, Daniel's brain wasn't quite right, possibly due to years of sleep deprivation. That's how it works. Poor sleep habits compromise your brain's functioning, and your dysfunctional brain can't recognize its own false normalcy. But everyone else does.

Why Sleep?

Sleep is a vital indicator of overall health and well-being. Like water and oxygen, it is necessary for your survival. During sleep, the nervous system performs critical functions. Growth hormones are released to provide proteins for cell growth and repair (hence the term "beauty sleep"). Memories and learning are encoded into the brain. Sleep is crucial for brain development in infants, and brain plasticity in adults. It directly affects hormone balance and weight management.

According to the National Sleep Foundation, adults need 7–9 hours of sleep consistently, more during times of illness or stress.

How can you MOVE IN THE DIRECTION OF more sleep?

Fortunately, sleep is governed by habits. Bad habits that work *against* you can be converted to good habits that work *for* you. You can turn around your poor sleep habits simply by (a) making a commitment and (b) making a plan. Implement your plan for one month, and your brain will adopt the new habits.

Make a Commitment

Changing your sleep habits will require you to change the way you do things, and you probably like the way you do things. These changes could affect others in your household, who may also like the way things are. Prepare for disruption. Until your new-and-improved sleep habits become the new norm, you'll need a strong "Why" to pull you past resistance to change.

> ✍ **Complete this sentence:**
> **The #1 reason I am committed to giving my body the sleep it needs is _________.**

Make a Plan

Make changes to eliminate any obstructive patterns. You may have to fight your brain on this step. Brains don't like change and create all sorts of excuses to resist it. Tell your brain to trust you. It, and you, can try anything for a month. Here are some changes you may consider (✓ Check off new habits you will implement):

- ☐ Eliminate sources of noise and light.
- ☐ Remove your clock. Use your cell phone's alarm.
- ☐ Remove your television. Watch TV in another room so that moving to the bedroom signals your brain that it's bedtime.
- ☐ Sequentially turn off lights as the evening progresses, until you are left with only a bedside lamp.
- ☐ Read from a book rather than a device or, at least, turn your device to a dark setting.
- ☐ Make your home quiet as bedtime nears.
- ☐ As you implement habits that support better sleep, wean yourself from sleep aids. They actually inhibit your brain's natural sleep cycle.
- ☐ No caffeine after 3 p.m.
- ☐ No exercise 1 hour prior to bedtime.
- ☐ Keep a notepad by the bed to download thoughts and worries.

✑ Write your plan to move in the direction of better sleep:
- **Goal**
- **Begin quiet time**
- **Desired time to bed**
- **Desired time up**
- **Pre-Sleep routine**
- **Handling disruptions**
- **Wake up routine**

Non-Negotiable #3: Moving the Body

If the gym is not your thing, putting it on your calendar 3 days a week is a setup for failure. It's not sustainable.

Yet, the body is designed to move. Some essential functions require the movement of muscles. Moving the body is a non-negotiable because without it, you compromise:

- Lymph function (immune support),
- Gene expression,
- Brain function (memory, cognitive ability, mood, stress-coping),
- Risk of developing neurodegenerative disorders,
- Optimum sexual function,
- Clearer skin,
- Sleep quality,
- Strong muscles, joints and bones.

We know the benefits of exercise, so why is it so hard? A study by the CDC estimates that 80% of American adults don't exercise. This is attributed to us being either too busy or too lazy. I think that is unkind. We are bombarded by very real pressures, time-demands, and disempowering commercial messaging like no other time in the history of mankind! We just can't handle—and don't think we deserve—one more thing, even if it is "good for us."

Let's just make this simple, sustainable and, even, fun. It doesn't have to be a big deal. Just move more. Make your body happy. Think about something you used to do for fun—dancing, skating, summersaults in the yard—and do that. Don't time it. Don't log it. Don't count calories.

How can you MOVE IN THE DIRECTION OF being more active?
Be more active today than you were yesterday. ⌂ Check-off activities you will try.

- ☐ Get a wearable tracker. Have fun tracking your progress. Engage in challenges with friends.
- ☐ Make a list: Activities I Enjoy.
- ☐ Download "50 Fun Ways to Get More Active TODAY" from www.LizGarrett.com/opposite
- ☐ Get a partner for accountability and fun.
- ☐ What did you enjoy doing when you were a child?
- ☐ Get on some equipment (stairstepper, elliptical trainer, treadmill) while you do something else. Multitasking is okay here.
- ☐ Sit less. Stand and walk more.

Non-Negotiable #4: Stress Management

Stress can serve us positively. It motivates us. It heightens awareness. It pushes us towards peak performance. Stress can increase your creativity. It compels us to reach higher. It tells you when there is something you need to change in your life. For all of these things, you can actually be grateful for stress.

Unmanaged, stress will kill us. Stress management is a non-negotiable for two reasons:

1. Stress involves a biological process that you can't override, is addictive, and damages your health.
2. Your ego thinks stress is a good thing and, unchecked, will allow the parasite (stress) to destroy the host (you). Warning: your clever ego may trick you into skipping this section, especially if you need it most.

Drug-Like Effect

Your body is made to respond to stress. When there is a loss of control, uncertainty, or conflict, your body floods itself with powerful neurotransmitters that prepare it for flight or fight: increasing heart rate, breathing, muscular response, and alertness, as well as stimulating adrenals for an energy boost which ultimately increases appetite and stores fat in your abdominal region.

This is a good thing if you do need to fight or run, but when it happens every day, all day, sitting in your office, that tightness and high level of responsiveness actually wears out your response system.

Stress is a buzz and it is addictive. You can't control the chemical response that occurs in your body. When it occurs repeatedly, it changes your neurology very much like drug or alcohol dependency. Stress is an addiction. Your response pathways, if exposed to stress over and over, became etched so that a stress-reaction is all your body knows to do, whether it is appropriate or not. The slightest trigger gets the exact same response as a major threat. The body can't tell the difference anymore. The adrenalin rush makes you feel protected in the moment but, in actuality, it is frying your brain power.

Chronic stress compromises your health in many, many ways. Constant stress shrinks a key memory center. Chronic stress gnaws on the little ends of your DNA so that your cells don't replicate correctly, aging you by up to ten years. Chronic stress, even small ongoing conflicts, increases the odds of stress-related illness three to five times.

It is in your body—the physiologic effect—where stress has the most unignorable and motivating effect. While your powerful mind may be able to hide from your awareness stress's negative effect on your general happiness, painful physical symptoms will drive you to seek change. See if you see yourself here . . .

✓ Which "red flags" are you experiencing?

   ☐ Fatigue

- ☐ High blood pressure
- ☐ Insomnia
- ☐ Increased occurrences of illness and infection
- ☐ Susceptibility to autoimmune disorders
- ☐ Gastrointestinal disorders
- ☐ Sexual dysfunction
- ☐ Irritability
- ☐ Reduced fertility
- ☐ Chronic headaches
- ☐ Mental impairment
- ☐ Inclination toward: overeating, alcohol abuse, smoking, couch potatoism, addiction
- ☐ More stress (it's a vicious cycle)

◎ Surround yourself with tools and reminders to beat stress.

How can you MOVE IN THE DIRECTION OF less stress? Check-off the strategies you might put into place.

- ☐ Know and prepare for your stressors – create the suggested table.
- ☐ Use deep-breathing.
- ☐ Use essential oils.
- ☐ The other non-negotiables—nutrition, sleep, activity and mindset—help you with stress.
- ☐ Use EFT (Emotional Freedom Technique).
- ☐ Meditate.
- ☐ Get organized.
- ☐ Take supplements, especially Vitamin B.
- ☐ Schedule and take breaks.
- ☐ Put a JFM (Just For Me) on your calendar every day.
- ☐ Laugh! Reach out to a funny friend or go to a funny website.

- ☐ Go on a Rampage of Appreciation.
- ☐ Talk it out—7 minute limit.
- ☐ Take a nap if you need one.
- ☐ Protect yourself from EMFs.
- ☐ Assume responsibility. Change what you can change to move out of victimhood.
- ☐ When feeling overwhelmed, review your agreements: renegotiate or cancel.

> 📄 **Foil stress before it even hits you! Have your Stress Prevention Plan ready--a reference table with these headings:**
> - **Key Stressor**
> - **Alternative Choice**
> - **Consequences of Alternative Choice**
> - **Dealing with Consequences**
>
> **Stress Prevention Plan form is downloadable at www. trueyouadvantage.com/opposite**

Non-Negotiable #5: Positive Mindset

Mindset is a non-negotiable because YOU ALREADY HAVE ONE. Your thoughts and beliefs are wired into your brain, forming neural networks through which every sensory input is processed. This creates your experience (positive or negative), expectations, abilities and limitations. Eventually, the mindset that got you where you are won't get you further, and will actually hold you back. You've reached that point if . . .

- ☐ You're not getting the raises or promotions you expect.
- ☐ Your personal relationships are not advancing.
- ☐ Your health is declining, perhaps in subtle ways.

- [ ] You can't get out of debt.
- [ ] Your dreams for your life seem continually out of reach.
- [ ] Words like "stuck," "trapped," "depressed," "overwhelmed," "confused," or "frustrated" regularly enter your mind and vocabulary.

Is your stinkin' thinkin' holding you back? Guess what! You programmed your brain, and you can re-program it at any time with a Mindset Reset!

Success is no secret. Just as anyone with the correct combination can open a lock, the Success Mindset is available to everyone. Just study the time-proven principles and practices successful people use. You can't do it alone. As Einstein told us, you can't solve a problem from the same level of consciousness that created it. Put another way, you can't know what you don't know. You need to look for resources outside yourself to reprogram your thinking.

How can you MOVE IN THE DIRECTION OF positive mindset?

In "The Success Principles," Jack Canfield provides 67 timeless principles and practices used by the world's most successful people. The first, foundational, Success Principle is "Assume 100% responsibility" for your life.

> ✎ **Where could you give up:**
> **Blaming? Complaining? Justifying?**
> **Defending? Excuse Making?**

You've got to claim it to change it, and this exercise from Jack Canfield will help:

✍ Difficult or Troubling Situation Exercise

1. What is a difficult or troubling situation in your life?
2. How are you creating it or allowing it to happen?
3. What are you pretending not to know?
4. What is the payoff for keeping it like it is?
5. What is the cost for not changing it? 6. What would you rather be experiencing?
6. What actions will you take and what requests will you make to get it?
7. By when will you take that action?
8. On a scale of 1-10 (10 being highest probability), will you follow through on this action?

Self Coaching: Self-Management

You've covered a lot of ground in this chapter. Let's chunk it down into actionable steps so you can gain traction before continuing to the next chapter. Remember, all you need to do is MOVE IN THE DIRECTION OF self-management. Get going now; you will revisit and make adjustments regularly.

Gift yourself some time to explore these questions with pen and paper:

1. What is your biggest obstacle to self-management? Now, take it 5 levels deep: Why? And Why? What else? Really, why?

2. What 3 actions appeal most to you?

3. What one action are you willing to double-dare commit to?

4. Circling back to your first answer, how will you support your success?

*Now that you've got a "vehicle" maintenance plan,
you get to decide what you're driving. Is it a Prius, a Jeep, or a
Maserati? In the next chapter, gain control over how people see and
treat you by developing your personal brand.*

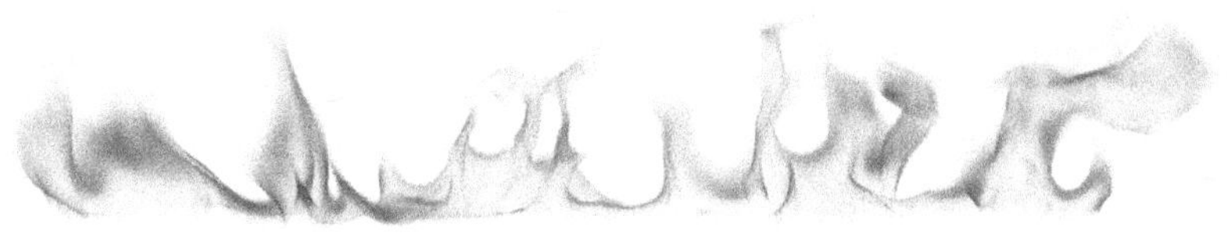

What you put out into the world comes back to you. How others see and treat you is determined, first, by how you see yourself. Use these tools and strategies to put your best into the world, so you'll get the best back.

Essential Strategy #2:

Personal Branding

PERSONAL BRANDING IS ABOUT PRESENTING yourself to others to engage them in what you want to accomplish: your mission. More evolved than its passive cousin, Reputation, Personal Branding is consciously developed. It comes from within, from your deepest, truest self. It drives your decisions. It enforces your boundaries. It weaves strategies to get what you want. It gives you a strong "why." Personal branding is founded on your life purpose or mission, and emanates through everything you do. Personal Branding is a valuable counter to burnout because it enables you to release the trivial b.s. that creates stress and subterfuge, while keeping you focused on what matters . . . to YOU.

The Essential Advantage

The workplace—or life, in general—can seem an endless gladiator-style competition. The battle to stay ahead of everyone in every way is unwinnable. The competition mindset is a setup for burnout. There is a better way. Recognize that your advantage is your uniqueness. By maximizing your individual talents, passions and perspectives, you make the most of what you have to offer on a single-player field. No one can compete to be the best you, except you!

Entrepreneurial Attitude

First, you must get that YOU are your product, your profit center, your commodity. Even if (especially if) you are employed by someone else, approaching your career with an entrepreneurial mindset keeps you in control.

Here's why:

- If you don't have a brand, the course of your work will be defined by someone else's brand.
- If you don't determine your value, someone else will.
- If you don't engage in work that fulfills you, you will crumble under the enormous and constant pressure to produce for someone else's benefit.

CEO of You, Inc.

Think like a CEO. What qualities do you want to be known for? What great successes do you want to achieve? What is your mission? What do you want to accomplish with your life's work? What is your business today? Who are your competitors? What will your "business" look like in five years? Ten years? What skills will be relevant in your business going forward? What investments will you make in yourself? What ROI (return on investment) do you expect to see?

✍ Conduct a SWOT Analysis

Strengths	**Weaknesses**
What unique abilities or experience do you offer?	*What skills or experience do you need but lack?*
Opportunities	**Threats**
What needs exist or are developing in your market?	*What conditions or occurrences could limit your success?*

Identify Your Mission Statement

Every strong company is guided by a mission statement, and You, Inc., is no different. You have the power to create the life you want, the career you want, so first you must get clear on exactly *what* you want.

We're not talking about an "Elevator Pitch," that pithy 30-second declaration you could use to fully enlighten a stranger. Those are externally focused, designed to affect or maybe manipulate said stranger. Your Mission Statement is internally focused. It is your compass for navigating the journey of your career. Whether or not you share your Mission Statement (in an elevator or elsewhere), it is in your mind and heart as you present yourself, make choices, and respond to opportunities.

"Mission" defined:

- It is not (necessarily) a vocation.
- It changes/morphs throughout life.
- It may be too obvious to see.
- It gives meaning to activity.

- It leverages your strengths.
- It is not (necessarily) sexy.
- It provides a framework for conscious choice.
- It is revealed in stages throughout life.
- It is essentially spiritual, not mental or physical.

What it means to "find it:"

- It's already in you, so the process is uncovering, not creating.
- Get aligned with your passions and your gifts.
- Take action in a direction and watch for signposts and feedback.
- It's not an endpoint.
- Become aware.
- Choose actions that support it.

Reinforcing signposts – Moving in the Direction of True You:

- Life is always expanding and opening up—there is WONDER.
- You see the lives of others benefiting from your life.
- You become aware of how all of life is purposeful.
- There is joy. (Joy is your GPS!)
- You have experiences of tapping into a bigger energy resource.
- You experience right-timing (synchronicities).
- You feel the presence of God (whatever you perceive the ever-present, creative source to be) more often.

Tools for Finding Your Mission Statement

Your Mission Statement is your personal brand. Don't worry if you think you haven't got a clue. You do! Here are some exercises to help you uncover your mission statement. It doesn't matter what age you are now—it is never too early or late to discover your mission, especially since it evolves over the course of your life.

List-Mining

- Previous achievements/accomplishments, and the talent, strength, or ability involved
- Qualities you admire in others (make a list of people and their qualities)
- Strengths embedded in weaknesses (make a list of your "faults" and the embedded talent or skill you value)
- Categories of Talent (make lists of your skills with people, your skills with physical things, and your skills with information)

> 📄 **These lists can help you uncover identifying personal talents that point to your unique mission.**

Life Review

- When you look back, are there any peak experiences that stand out?
- Are there activities you enjoy so much you lose all sense of time?
- What were your childhood passions?
- Imagine looking back from the end of your life (retirement, eulogy, etc). What do you want to have accomplished?

Jack Canfield's Mission Statement Exercise

1. Identify two of your unique personal qualities, such as enthusiasm and creativity (adjectives).

2. Identify one or two ways you most enjoy expressing those qualities when interacting with others (verbs).

3. Describe the world as you would like to see it if it were perfect right now. How is everyone interacting with everyone else? What does it feel like? Remember, a perfect world is a fun place to be.

4. Combine the three prior statements into a single statement:

[My Qualities] + [What I Do] = So That [Outcome]

Consult the Experts

1. Make a list of 10 people who know you, who you respect and admire.

2. Personally contact each with this question: What are 3 unique ways I contribute value?

> ✍ **Get off Go with your Mission Statement.
> Write it down, knowing it will refine and
> evolve as you move through life with it.**

Make Your Mission Your Brand

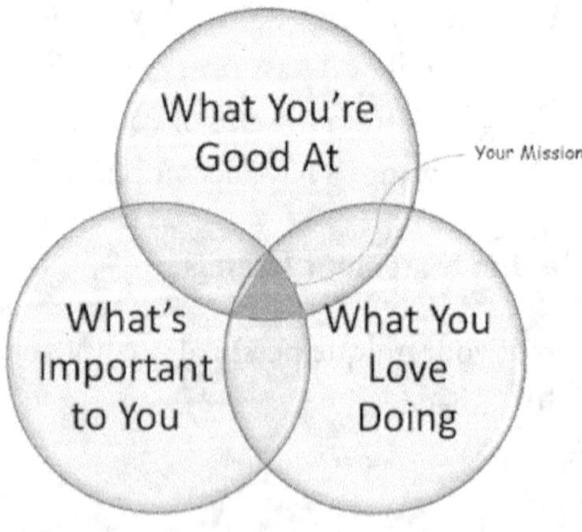

Being clear about what you're good at, what you love doing, and what's important to you gives you an advantage against burnout. Just that awareness, alone, begins to direct your efforts and inform your choices. You can't unknow what you know, and if you know what makes your heart sing, you won't be able to deny it very long. Sooner or later you'll have to bring it into your life.

This doesn't necessarily mean quitting your job and working in a soup kitchen! Your best strategy weaves together the *qualities* of your mission statement with the valued skills gained from your education and experience. It's not mission _or_ job, it's both. Your job creates the means and opportunity to realize your mission.

Your brand is how you express your mission to the world. It's what you're about. It's what you're on earth to accomplish. It's your growth path. It's how everyone sees you. It's what you live for.

▤ Put Your Brand into Action

1. **Make a list of 10 qualities that are associated with your mission. These may be things like: dependable, compassionate, strong, creative, good writer, etc.**

2. **Convert each quality to an affirmation by putting the words "I am" in front of it. Tweak the wording so it makes sense and rings true.**

3. **For each affirmation, develop a way to demonstrate it to the world.**

4. **Review your list of affirmations several times daily. Keep it handy in your planner, in your car, in your pocket, by your bed, on your desk. Memorize it.**

Job Crafting

Once you are clear on your mission, your work becomes a platform to accomplish your mission. Seek points of alignment between your employer's mission and your own. Step up to opportunities that allow you to demonstrate your brand. What you focus on, increases, so focus on tasks and objectives that give you energy and keep you engaged. Put your attention and energy on creating more opportunities to do what you're good at, what you love doing, and what's important to you, and your job will morph into perfection.

Here's a great example of job crafting. A woman worked in health & safety at a major industrial site, but she loved cats and longed to find a profession that would pay well and involve cats. Good luck with that, right?! Through the process of identifying her mission and branding herself as a cat-lover, she was able to implement a program to manage the feral cat population on her job site. This was formalized as a health & safety objective and added to her job description . . . with an increase in pay!

Passion Projects

What would you do if you won the lottery? A kaleidoscope of possibilities just flashed before your eyes, probably things like travel, houses, cars, sleep. And then what? If you didn't have to worry about money, is there something you would do simply because it's important to you? That's a Passion Project. And you don't have to win the lottery to make it happen.

Consider bringing your brand, your talents, your energy and your resources to a specific project that excites you, inspires you and satisfies you. Passion Projects can be:

- Long-term or short-term;
- Within work or outside of work;

- Something you do on the weekends or evenings;
- A professional goal.

Reflection as a Tool

To combat extremely high rates of burnout among medical professionals, Loyola University Chicago Stritch School of Medicine teaches students to use reflection as a fundamental tool to prevent burnout. Students carry a small notebook in their lab coat to write answers to reflection questions, including:

- What surprised you?
- What touched you?
- What inspired you?
- Do you feel you are becoming the professional you wish to be?

The Upward Spiral

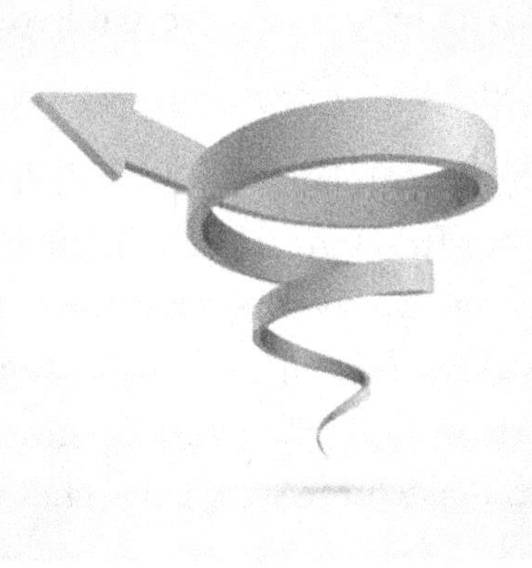

Your brand—your mission—will continually evolve. Once you put it out into the world, you will get feedback to help you gain greater clarity. Some of that feedback will feel positive (raises, accolades, appreciation), and some of it will feel negative (disapproval, setbacks, failure). Either way, see it for what it is: just feedback. Ultimately, it is not the events of your life that determine your experience; it your response to those events.

There is always this invisible line. Above it is positive, uplifting, strengthening. Below it is negative, depressing, weakening. Both exist at all times. Neither is more or less "real" than the other. There is no neutral. Everything has an energetic charge, one pole or the other.

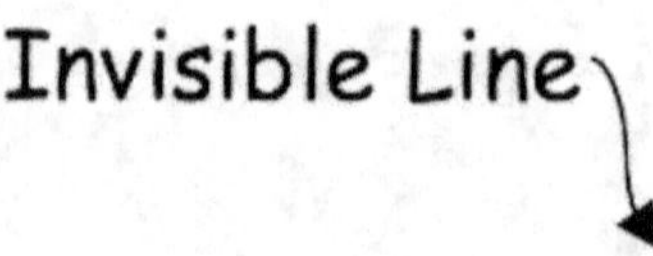

In every choice, in every moment, you are always moving things in an upward or downward direction. This is the simple and empowering concept of the Upward Spiral: your health, finances, happiness—every aspect of your life—are getting better or worse in every microsecond, depending on where you choose to direct your focus.

Your choices and habits accumulate, compound, and gain momentum in the direction you choose. This is great news! With any moment, with even the tiniest choice, you can change the direction of your life toward your mission. Then, as these little incremental changes build upon themselves, you get stronger and stronger, your brain ingrains the new habit, and it gets easier and easier to make more supportive choices that point your life upward.

You are caught in a self-perpetuating spiral of experience, upward or downward. Your moment of power is when you remember the Invisible Line, and decide what your experience will be!

**🔔 *RIGHT NOW*, ask yourself if there are areas
of your life that are trending downward? How will you
reverse the direction today? Make it a habit to remember
the power of
the upward spiral as you make choices.**

Self Coaching: Personal Brand

Write your mission statement here:

If your Mission Statement were an outfit,
    How would it feel?
    What colors would it be?
    How would people describe you in it?
How will you honor and celebrate your mission?

- ☐ Share it (With whom? Where?)

- ☐ Create art or Vision Board

- ☐ Put it on website and social media

- ☐ Create branded clothing or jewelry

- ☐ Post it in workspace

- ☐ Read affirmations daily

---

*Awesome! You've got a mission statement
and are clear on your brand. You're ready to make a
difference in the world! In the next chapter you'll gain satisfying tools
and strategies to help you get it all done.*

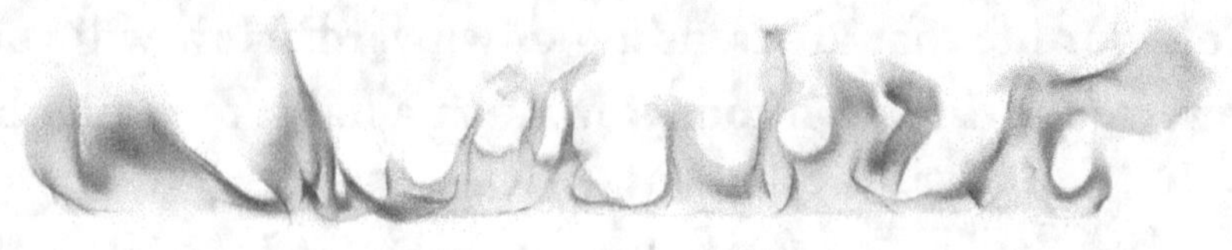

Essential Strategy #3:

Mindful Organization

WHEN INSIDES DON'T MATCH OUTSIDES, there is friction. Think of that friction as fueling the fire of burnout. Let's reduce the friction by making sure the way you use your space, time and actions reflects your best self and highest potential. *Mindful* organization goes beyond arbitrary neatness and efficiency. *Mindful* organization consciously leverages your space, time and tasks to launch you toward your idea of success with greater ease and joy. *Mindful* organization is strategic and purposeful, and very, very personal.

This is not a book on organization (although you should get one). This is a book about living your life according to your terms and priorities so you can enjoy a long, fruitful career. You're going to need to develop and maintain mindfulness in three pervasive dimensions: Space, Time and Tasks.

What does "mindful" mean?

Living in alignment with your priorities requires you to put a keen "eyeball of awareness" on all you do, what fills your space, and what you give your time to, with increasing demand that everything support, not undermine, your goals and mission. Mindfulness can get brutal. Once you tune in, you will naturally favor that which supports your personal priorities and release that which does not. This means you will have to let go of some habits, possessions and people that hold you back. This can be painful, and often involves time and grieving. Distraction will tempt you to take the easier road. Be gentle.

The First Dimension: Time

Stop with "Too Busy"

"Busy" is <u>not</u> a good thing. Here's what feeling, thinking and saying you're "too busy" says about you:

- You're unskilled in managing your time.
- You say "yes" when you should say "no."
- You value other people's respect, pity and/or approval more than your own well-being.
- You are unaware that everyone gets the same 24 units of time per day.
- You don't value your time (so why should anyone else?).

Stop wearing "Busy" like a badge of honor. There is no pride in busy-ness. Busy-ness compromises productivity and results. Busy-ness is a function of priorities, not time. Busy-ness sends the message that you are in over your head. Busy-ness is creating stress. Nearly *half of employees (47%)* polled by LifeCare said "time management" was the number one source of stress in their lives.

> 🔔 **Today: Notice how often the word "busy" enters your mind and exits your mouth.**

Get Real About the Grid of Time

Learn to view your time objectively as 24 blocks. It's finite. Pretending otherwise gives you the false impression that you can do everything. You can't. You can do anything, but not everything. Time management is really priority management.

Make it tangible. Put everything on your calendar so you can see it and manage it within the grid of time. Recognize distortions. Your energy levels, likes/dislikes, and wishful thinking alter your perception of time.

Get Real About Time Requirements

When scheduling, err on the side of too much. Factor in hidden time requirements like interruptions, setup, cleanup, research, and travel. Record how long tasks and events actually took. Review your calendar objectively: Does your use of time align with your priorities? Show me your calendar and I'll tell you your truth.

Commit to Your Calendar

Your mindset around your calendar is one of your biggest indicators of sustainable success. Here's what *doesn't* work:

- "I don't need a calendar. I can remember my appointments."
- "My calendar says x, but I'll do y."
- "I never look at my calendar."
- "I'm not sure I wrote that down right." ("So I'll just guess at it.")
- "Let me check my other calendars."
- "There is no time for exercise/social time/vacation/etc."
- "Sorry I'm late." ("I didn't schedule adequate time for travel and preparation.")

Not only do statements like those reflect badly on your competence, they set you up for a cycle of failure. Your commitment to your calendar is a matter of integrity that programs your brain. Here's how your brain sees it:

→ If you don't honor what's on your calendar, your brain ignores your calendar.

→ Once your brain ignores your calendar, it stops using its massive problem-solving ability to make things happen, and instead worries about your appointments.

Routinely disrespecting items on your calendar (like appointments to go to the gym, or to leave work by 5) tell your brain you aren't serious about those commitments and your brain need not put energy into bringing them to fruition. It's better to not make commitments you won't keep.

Think of your calendar as your commitment document. Fully commit to it. Conversely, don't add items you're not committed to. Write time-based activities in one place: appointments, calls, errands, chores. Review it regularly. Are your priorities well-represented? What do you want to add to your schedule? Remove? Are there commitments you regularly violate?

Paper or Digital?

There are advantages to both formats. Paper calendars appeal to more senses (visual, tactile) and engage more of your creative right-brain.

Digital calendars give you more power and depth. This is a matter of personal choice. Do what feels good, and when it no longer feels good, change it. You can change formats throughout your life. There is a hybrid option: keep your calendar digitally and print it out for tactile, visual interaction.

> ◎ **Download Tips for Mindful Organizing with Microsoft Outlook (M.O./M.O.) from www. TrueYouAdvantage.com/opposite.**

The Multitasking Myth

Neuroscientists have shown that the brain is not equipped to concentrate on two things simultaneously. The brain actually slows down when made to perform two mental tasks at the same time. It takes 64 seconds to retrieve train of thought after email interruption. Checking your email every five minutes means you are losing 8.5 hours per week (Thomas Jackson, PhD, Loughborough University). Want to uncover a full day each week? Refrain from checking email frequently.

More importantly, multitasking denies you the full experience of the task at hand, and begs the question, "Why are you doing things you don't want to be present for?" The phrase for this is "absent presence."

> 🔔 **If you catch yourself multitasking, consider it a red flag. Are you really working on *your* priorities?**

Time is Not Created Equal

Throughout the day, your energy and focus levels naturally fluctuate through 4 identifiable states. You can control some of the factors that influence the duration and frequency of these Time States (the 5 Non-Negotiables, for example), but you cannot "make yourself" achieve or sustain the higher Time States simply because you've got a deadline or specific schedule.

Time-State	Characterized by...	Best used for...
A-Time	...intense creativity and the perception of warped time; aka Flow State.	...highest priority mid-work, problem-solving, project development, creative expression.
B-Time	...strong productivity.	...cranking through tasks, email, meetings, To-Do list.
C-Time	...low mind engagement but still physically engaged	...exercise, house work, socializing.
D-Time	...low physical and mental engagement, heading toward exhaustion.	...activities that consciously restore mind and body.

Ride the Time States like a wave for maximum productivity and creativity. Here are 2 key strategies for maximizing Time States:

1. **Don't waste higher Time States on lower activities.**
   Reserve your A- and B-Times for your highest priorities. For example, if mornings are your A-time, get to work early and

schedule your workout and social time for later in the day. Vice-versa if your natural rhythms tend toward Night Owl.

2. **Don't force higher activities into lower Time States.**
   When A-Time has subsided, staring at your computer won't bring it back. Rather than forcing out subpar work you'll end up re-doing anyway, move on to a Time-State appropriate activity.

The Second Dimension: Space

Space Relations

You know how some rooms just make you feel good, and some rooms just feel yucky? It's a fact: the space around you affects you energetically. It either charges and supports you, or depletes and undermines you. Let's use this to your advantage. Use this awareness to consciously and methodically change your space to be what you need it to be.

Your relationship with the space you occupy is ongoing and dynamic. You change, your needs change, so the space needs to change. When it begins to get messy or feel bad, it's time to ask yourself "What's not working here?" and make the necessary changes to keep it in alignment with your brand.

Mindful management of the Space Dimension involves <u>consciousness</u> and <u>communication</u>.

Who's Telling Your Secrets?

Your non-verbals are SCREAMING . . . do you hear them? Everyone else does. Studies show non-verbal communication outweighs verbal communication. This is far more than body language. The appearance of your desk, car, office and home tells people:

- Whether or not you can be trusted with more opportunity;
- How much you respect yourself (and if they should respect you);
- How well you organize thoughts (associated with intelligence);
- How approachable you are.

Give some thought to the messages you send via the space you occupy, and make sure it is in alignment with your brand.

Define Your Vision for Each Space

Make a list of the places you find yourself in the course of a day. This may include: bedroom, bathroom, kitchen, living room, car, office, conference room, breakroom. For each space you occupy, answer 2 questions:

1. How can this space best support me? Depending on your intention for the space, some things to consider could include: comfort, inspiration, resources, quiet, etc.
2. What do I want this space to tell other people? This could include your interest and hobbies, accomplishments, goals, and passion project, as well as qualities you value such as focus, discipline, openness, intelligence, creativity, etc.

For shared space, the visioning process necessitates a discussion. Ask for a meeting or an agenda item on the next group meeting. Share these guidelines:

- Establish a basic premise: this process is for the benefit all involved (win-win).
- Respect others' needs as well as your own.
- Don't make it personal.
- Speak in terms of "us," our," and "mine," not "yours."

> **📄 Agenda for Room Function Discussion**
>
> - **Current function**
> - **Ideal Function**
> - **Who uses it?**
> - **Who should/could us it?**
> - **What should it contain?**
> - **What needs to be removed?**
> - **Distribute an agenda in advance.**

Clutter

Clutter deserves special scrutiny. The tendency toward clutter is self-sabotaging and can indicate self-esteem issues. Clutter—or any form of space dysfunction—begs these questions:

- Do you feel unworthy of success?
- Do you want to create barriers between you and others?
- What truth do you need to see/admit/understand/address/heal?
- What do you need to change (inside or outside)?

Clutter is different from dirty or disorganized. Clutter is the accumulation of things you no longer even see, but which obstruct your productivity.

Clutter reduces your available space. Clutter makes people doubt your ability. Clutter adds stress and wastes time. The average U.S. executive wastes one hour per day searching for missing information in messy desks and files, according to a Wall street Journal article. This is over two weeks per year—what could you do with 2 weeks?

CHIP AWAY AT CLUTTER
Schedule 1 hour a day to address clutter.
Apply mindfulness. Watch for avoidance and distraction.
What truth does clutter need you to embrace?

The Third Dimension: Tasks

Mindful management of tasks means having a system that (a) captures tasks and (b) informs your choice to do tasks based on *your* available time, energy and priority. Lacking such a system puts you in a position to accomplish tasks based on other people's priority, without regard to your time and energy. That's a setup for burnout.

The Capture Process

The first step to bringing mindfulness to your tasks is to determine what those tasks are. If it's in your head, let it out! You'll experience instant relief and clarity, while freeing your brain for more important functions. Put your tasks into your organizing system so that you can see them objectively and manage them according to time, energy and priority. Tasks are most actionable when defined by desired outcomes and contain a verb.

🔔 On a regular basis, perform a
thorough inventory (a.k.a Mental
Dump) for each area of responsibility.

Resist the Tyranny of the To Do List

Make sure you run your lists, and your lists do not run you. As fulfilling as it feels to check things off your list, checking the *wrong* things off your list will lead you down the road of burnout. Your lists are for *reference*, to capture the results of a thought process, and to help you avoid reinventing the wheel every time you make a decision. Keeping To Do lists (a.k.a. Action Lists, Task Lists) keeps your mind clear. Acting on your To Do list should bring you satisfaction. This requires mindfulness.

You are the boss of your lists. Not the other way around.

Managing Tasks

Once you have a carefully culled list of tasks that represents your priorities and commitments, think about how you're managing those Tasks.

- Tasks become reality when place on your grid of time (your calendar).
- Stay aware of your priorities. This is not about getting as many things done as possible. It is about productively accomplishing the things that matter most to you.
- Determine activity according to your time-state and conscious priority, not someone else's sense of urgency.
- Organize tasks by what you value. This is where those reference lists come in handy, especially your Top 5 priorities, Mission Statement, and Goals.
- Remember, the whole point is to enjoy your day!

The Stephen Covey Way

You may (or may not; see The David Allen Way, below) want to prioritize these tasks to gain awareness and control over them. Stephen Covey, author of *The Seven Habits of Highly Effective People* and *First Things First* gave us the Time Management Matrix for prioritizing tasks. It classifies tasks based on urgency and importance to determine the tasks so you can decide your priorities.

Quadrant I Urgent and Important

- Includes crises, pressing problems, deadlines.
- May indicate urgency addiction.
- These tasks take care of themselves (at the expense of Quadrant II tasks).

Quadrant II Important but Not Urgent

- Includes preparation, prevention, values clarification, planning, relationship building, true re-creation, and empowerment.
- This is where you want to focus.
- Time invested here reduces Quadrant I.

Quadrant III Urgent but Not Important

- Includes interruptions, some phone calls/mails/reports/meetings, and many popular activities.
- These tasks are usually other people priorities, and/or have ego payoff.

Quadrant IV Not Urgent, Not Important

- Includes busywork, time wasters, escape activities.
- These tasks can be categorically eliminated.

Covey Matrix

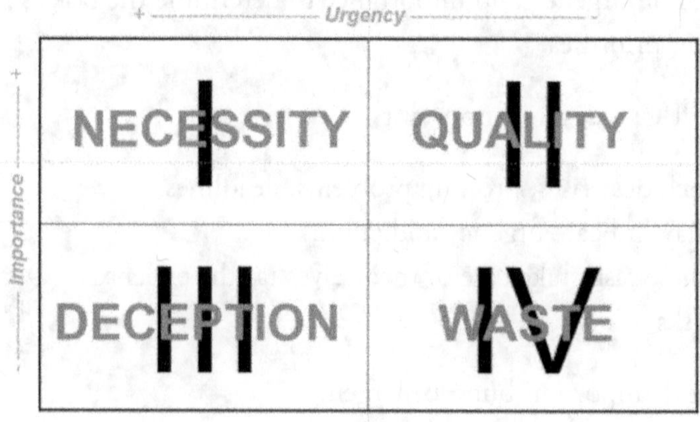

Steven R. Covey, *First Things First*

The David Allen Way

Instead of prioritizing tasks, advocates of the "Getting Things Done" (GTD) methodology, developed by David Allen, aspire for "mind like water." In this state, the mind is clear and free to respond appropriately to whatever stimuli come. Don't be fooled by its simplicity. GTD is as much a philosophical treatise as How To manual. It took me two years to begin to feel competent. After a decade of use, I continue to learn.

5 Stages of Workflow

GTD defines five distinct work phases. They are sequential and discrete. You can only do one at a time. Everything you do to the stuff in your life falls into these actions:

1. **Collect**—Identifying everything that has some potential action associated; recognize all your collection points; dump your mind.

2. **Process**—Getting In to empty; Asking What is This? Touching it Once. More than Checking, less than responding.
3. **Organize**—Where tasks are processed into your SYSTEM (lists, calendar, reference, delegation).
4. **Review**—Keeps you focused on your priorities; there are daily, weekly, and bigger picture reviews.
5. **Do**—Making the best action choices by time available and personal energy level.

How Will You Manage Your Tasks?

A successful organizing system has all of these qualities:

- You like using it.
- You can have it with you at all times.
- You trust it.
- You can adjust it as you evolve or your needs change.
- It frees you for productive creativity.

✓ **Optimize your task management**
Launch one approach (Covey, GTD or other) now and see where it takes you.
Be open. Be curious. Be consistent.

Self Coaching: Mindful Organization

1. What are your favorite distractions? What triggers them? What would help you switch back?

2. What do you want less of on your calendar? More of?

3. What steps will you take immediately to elevate the energy of your space?

4. What works in your Task Management approach? What needs to change?

Doesn't it feel GREAT to know you are spending your precious time and energy on what's important . . . to you?! The next chapter shows you how to make your priorities important to other people, too.

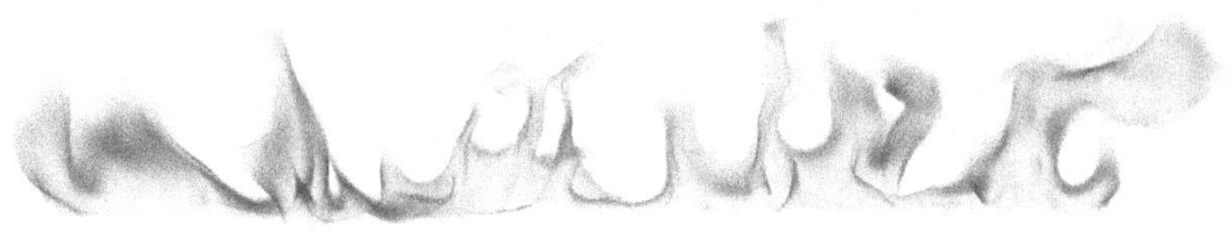

Essential Strategy #4:

Smart Communication

COMMUNICATION SKILLS ARE YOUR #1 promotability factor, more important than your education, experience, popularity, ambition or tenacity (*Harvard Business Review*). Although the majority of their work involves some form of communication, very few professionals invest time and effort into developing communication skills, defaulting, instead, to the skill level they learned early in life. "Goo goo gah gah," only gets you so far. Set yourself apart with smart communication skills that:

- Build alliances,
- Focus on specific desired outcomes,
- Strategize at least 3 steps out,
- Give up "Being Right" in favor of "Being Effective,"

- Get you more of what you want so you beat burnout.

Employers Love Great Communicators

Here are the Top 10 Communication Skills for Workplace Success (Alison Doyle, *The Balance*):

> **Put these concepts into action:**
> 🗎 **Put a star beside the qualities and skills you need to develop now.**
> 🔔 **Work these qualities into your day by writing them into your planner.**

1. Listening – Listening is your power position. Imagine your power leaking out of you every time you talk. Listening builds relationships. Listening resolves problems. Listening gives you information. Stephen Covey wrote, "Seek first to understand, and then to be understood."

2. Nonverbal communication – Creating alignment between you message and your non-verbal communication amplifies your effectiveness and reinforces your brand. Be conscious of the many ways you communicate nonverbally: tone of voice, word choice, the position of your body, clothing, jewelry, habits, facial expressions, vocal sounds, appearance, posture, and many, many more. Everything about you is a form of non-verbal communication.

3. Clarity and concision – Speak and write in soundbites: short, carefully-crafted messages that pack a punch and get remembered and repeated. Long, rambling messages that use big words don't make you look smarter, gain respect, or compel your listener to take action.

4. Friendly tone – Build a smile into your voice to convey respect and interest. People will want to hear what you have to say.
5. Confidence – You weren't born knowing how to speak. It is a craft you must learn and practice. Find a Toastmasters chapter near you.
6. Empathy – Putting yourself in another's shoes with compassion and grace doesn't make you weak; it makes you desired team player. What you say about other people says more about you than them.
7. Open-Mindedness – A willingness to see other people's side establishes you as an effective leader.
8. Respect – Manners matter! Learn and use proper business etiquette as it pertains to eye contact, greetings, meetings, and communication. These rules continually change as the work environment continually changes—keep up.
9. Feedback – Everyone is in a position to give and receive feedback. Treating it like the gift it is shows employers that you understand your role as a team player.
10. Picking the right medium – Texting, IMing, emailing, phoning, meeting—which is right? It's not about you—it's about your listener. Be able to use the appropriate communication medium to convey your message effectively. Stay current in the constantly evolving realm of "netiquette."

Social Component

Social support is the largest predictor of success or failure. Burnout does not occur in a vacuum. While you have your head down, hard at work, conditions around you may be setting you up for burnout. Think about it: your burnout—fully exhausting you as a fuel source—serves others at your detriment. Becoming aware of this, and exerting some control and influence over your social environment, are crucial for career sustainability.

❧ You are the sum of the 5 people you spend the most time with. Do they lift you up or bring you down? Write their names across the "5 Closest People" chart below (downloadable at http://www.TrueYouAdvantage. com/opposite), and put + or − beside each category.

	Name	Name	Name	Name	Name
You feel good when you're with them.					
You learn from them or discussions you have with them.					
They help you be a better person.					
You admire them, their success and/or happiness.					
You are unguarded and authentic in their company.					
ESTIMATED TIME SHARED WEEKLY					
GOAL TIME SHARED WEEKLY					

I'm not suggesting you cut anyone out of your life. I am suggesting you take 100% responsibility for how much time you give to whom. Take a close look at your reasons for keeping "-" people in your top 5. If it is any of the following, recognize that you are allowing your life to be pulled downward for ego gratification. You must decide if the payoff is worth the cost.

- ☐ Obligation
- ☐ Guilt
- ☐ Convenience
- ☐ Habit

☐ Misery loves company

Your relationships are moving you upward or downward on the energetic spiral—there is no neutral. Apply the "moving in the direction of" principle to the people you share your precious time with.

The more +s in their column, **expand** your time with them. Make them a priority. Proactively schedule time with them.

The more –s in their column, **contract** your time with them. Make meetings as short as possible. Put off scheduling time with them as long as possible. They can still be in your life, but not in the top 5 people you spend time with.

Another option is to begin to **transform the relationship**. You have full control over your behaviors and your speech. Don't engage in negative talk, complaining or gossip. Rather than responding, even if that's what you've always done, meet undesired "downward spiral" statements with silence. See what fills the void.

The Approval Trap

Each of your relationships exists in a dynamic tension that keeps you static relative to the other. It's a dance with both partners keeping tension on a rope between them. They move, you move. You move, they move. The tacitly agreed upon level of tension must be maintained. When you decide to change your moves—advance, grow, change—the other (usually unconsciously) applies tension to keep you in the same ol' dance. Since you like, respect, and/or even love the person, you (also unconsciously) want to make them happy. This works for both of you, until it doesn't.

Signs that it's working for them, but not you:

- You are fearful or concerned about their reaction to your change.
- The possibility (or threat) of their disapproval controls your behavior.
- They overtly or covertly block your growth and development.

Get used to this: saving yourself from burnout will piss some people off. You are in a fight for your life—it's them or you. This is your opportunity to improve the relationship by bringing your truth to it.

Three ways to help others deal with your change:

- Reassure them with this message frequently: "It's not against you, it's for me."
- Have and assume positive intent. Give them the benefit of the doubt.
- Broken record: repeat the same message over and over with same words, same tone. You'll know they've heard you when they repeat it back like it was their idea.

Stick with it! With persistence and consistency, you will bring the change you need to so that you can thrive. The result of your commitment to your needs will be a new dynamic tension that works for *you*.

Authentic Communication

Communicate to relate, not manipulate. Because authentic communication broadcasts vulnerability, respect, and truth, it creates connection. Connection creates sustainable success.

Authentic communication is not a permission slip to whine, gripe, complain, slack, grumble, yell, cry or puke negativity in any form on those around you. It is the opposite. Authentic communication is a responsibility. At every moment you have a wide array of "truths" to choose from. Remember the invisible line? Choose to convey a message that conveys the best version of True You.

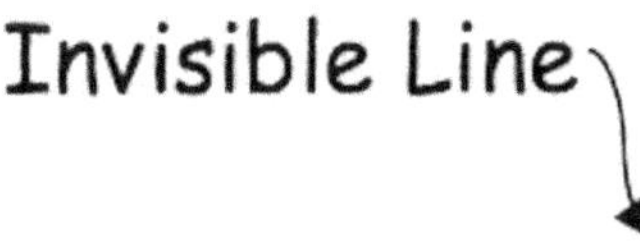

Guidelines for authentic communication (From Susan Campbell's "Getting Real: 10 Truth Skills You Need to Live an Authentic Life"):

1. Create a connection before speaking.
2. Speak from your own experience. Use "I" statements.
3. Know your intent: is it to control or relate?
4. Share your here-and-now experience (your thoughts and feelings).
5. Give feedback with this formula, "When you X, I felt/thought Y . . ."
6. If you are judging someone, own it and name it.
7. If you are making an interpretation about someone, own it and name it.
8. Keep checking in on your body's reaction.
9. Speak only when it feels right or you want to speak.
10. Be honest in your listening.

Influencing People

The Platinum Rule®

Maybe you know the Golden Rule: do unto others as you want done to you. Dr. Tony Alessandra teaches the Platinum Rule®: Do unto others as THEY want done unto them. For others to receive and act on your message, you must giftwrap it in their style, values and priorities.

There are a number of behavioral/personality models available. Choose the one you like, learn it, and include it in your tool chest. DISC is a good one. DISC is a behavior assessment tool developed by industrial psychologist Walter Vernon Clarke, based on the theory of psychologist William Moulton Marston.

> ✍ **Write in the names of people you work and/or live with, including your own.**

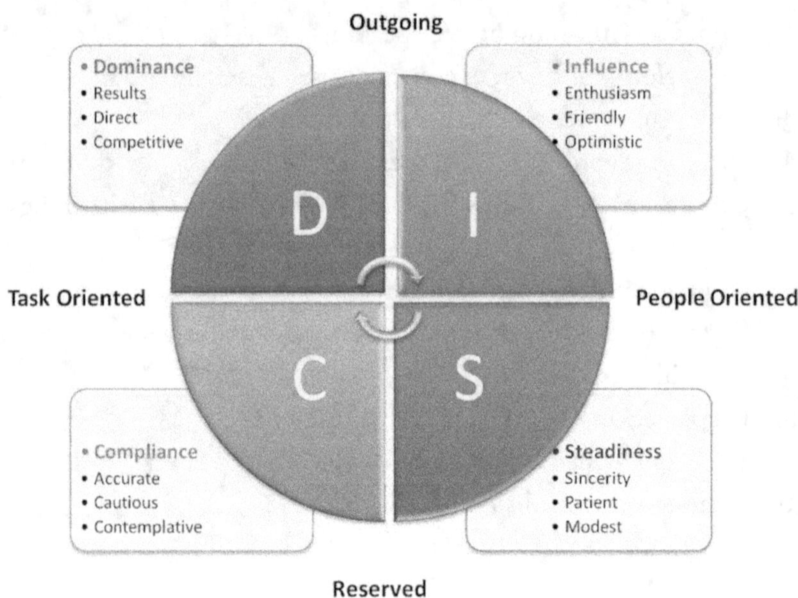

The importance of understanding behavioral styles is:

- Recognize your own style and how people perceive you.
- Use caution with people whose behavioral style is opposite yours.

- Modify your communication style in order to be successful with people.

When you are communicating with a D, speak in bullet points and bottom line.

When you are communicating with an I, be positive and oriented toward involvement.

When you are communicating with a S, develop a personal connection first.

When you are communicating with a C, give data/input to support a process.

Winning Work

In business, you eat what you kill. If you think that sounds harsh, someone has been feeding you. If you are thinking, "Oh YEAH, Bring it on, babycakes!" then you are hungry. Hungry is good! If you want to continue to eat indefinitely, learn how to win work. Winning work gives you more control over what projects you will work on. Winning work increases your personal credibility and job security. Winning work can make you rich.

Winning work requires you to absolutely master three skillsets you probably weren't taught in school:

1. Writing skills – grammar, succinctness, style, persuasion
2. Presenting skills – techniques to deliver complicated ideas in a way that provokes positive action
3. Networking skills – a keen understanding of the nuances of political and social interaction

Invest in developing these skills. Your ROI: the professional with the best skills wins (work)!

Being a Leader

A leader is a leader 24/7/365/∞. Eyes are always upon you: when you are buying coffee at the corner market; when you are passing people in the hallway; when you are at your kid's soccer game. You establish yourself as a leader long before people actually follow you.

A leader is a leader regardless of position. A job title does not automatically confer the power of leadership, nor does lack of a job title preclude it.

A leader is, by definition, out in front. A leader is willing to take risks because they've built connections and know their team has their back.

Guidelines for non-verbal communication that gains respect as a leader:

- Develop and project quiet confidence. Confident people convey authority.
- Maintain 30-36" personal space in workplace conversations.
- Face the person you're speaking to.
- Center your body. Don't lean.
- Put yourself at eye level or slightly above the person you're speaking with.
- Move slowly and purposefully—don't hurry.
- Have straight but relaxed posture.
- Lean toward people to show interest.
- Smile.
- Use natural gestures.
- Maintain proper eye contact (3-7 secs at a time).
- Dress a step above. Dress for the job you want.
- Consistently convey respect and interest in others.

Do you strive to be a fair-minded manager? Know this: there is a special burnout that strikes fair-minded managers. According to a study in the *Journal of Applied* Psychology, their commitment to procedural fairness, suppressing personal biases, and providing support and consistency to subordinates is a sure path to burnout. Managing the perceptions of subordinates during times of ambiguity and uncertainty can be a very draining. Recognize that being a successful fair-minded manager must be coupled with an unshakable commitment to extreme self-management.

Saying "No"

Reasons why you need to say "No" frequently:

- Every "yes" you give says "no" to something else (probably self-care and loved-ones).
- Saying "yes" frequently completely devalues your "yes." No one respects it.
- If you don't live by your own priorities, others will use you for their priorities.
- Saying "yes" when you can't actually give your best is selfish and impedes the other person's progress.
- Your task list will be shorter and you will be more effective and joyful.

Set your default response to requests to "hesitation." Be ruthless about only accepting tasks that are in alignment with your values and priorities. Equate accepting a task to making a commitment; if you can't commit, don't say "yes." Jack Canfield teaches the "Hell Yes" Test. If you don't feel resounding excitement about the request being made of you, seriously consider declining it.

Here is a formula for saying "No." Adapt it to fit your style or situation.

Step 1: Repeat the request. Ask clarifying questions. Take time with this step for two important reasons: you're increasing the value of what's being requested, and you're assuring the requester you understand the request (so there is no wiggle room in your "No").

Step 2: Turn them down while still offering a solution to their problem. You may:

- Suggest another person who is better suited
- Suggest another time-frame which works for you
- Suggest something different
- Just say "No." "No" is a complete sentence. Some other ways to say "No" include:
  - o "I won't be able to do that."
  - o "That won't work for me."
  - o "I understand the importance of what you're asking. Here is how I can help . . ."
  - o "I can't help you this time. Next time (give me more lead time, send a meeting request, whatever) . . ."

Do you notice what is missing from the formula? There is no apology! You have a right to decline a request—no apology is needed. Be greedy with your apologies. Save them for actual mistakes. Don't devalue them by throwing them around when you aren't really sorry.

What about saying "No" to your boss? When your boss makes a request you need to decline, adjust the formula slightly. Step 1 remains the same. Change Step 2 to this: "You're asking me to do this (state the request). My priorities for today were these (list them out). What is most important to you?"

🔔 Practice saying "No" in low-risk situations before you whip it out at work.

SPIRAL Into Better Communication

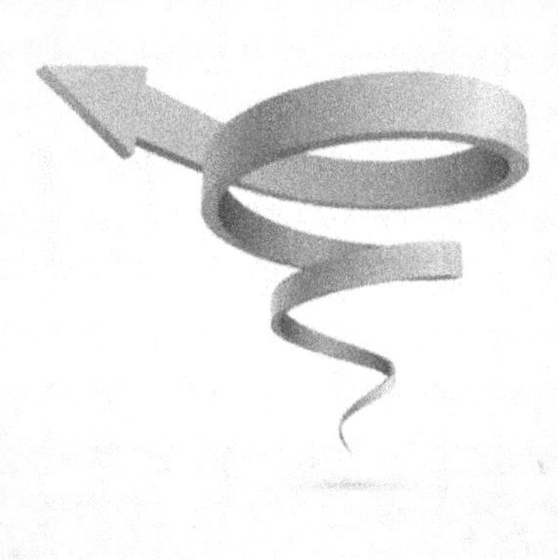

Here's a memory hook to help you remember the Upward Spiral as a tool for turning around even the toughest communication encounters:

Stop – Zip the lip. Take a breath. Still and relax the body.

Process – As objectively as possible, get clear about what is really happening, especially your contribution to the difficulty.

Invisible line – In any micro-moment, you are choosing UP (positive, uplifting, strengthening) or DOWN (negative, depressing, weakening). Find a way to pivot UP.

Reach for tools – Look for support and resources outside yourself. The consciousness that created the problem cannot solve the problem.

Authentic – Whatever is happening, lean in to your truth. No faking!

Learn, learn, learn – Every experience contains the gift of a lesson. It is up to you to receive and apply it.

Self Coaching: Smart Communication

1) What's your plan for improving your relationships? Include person, actions you'll take and desired outcome.

2) What work would you LOVE to win?

3) What will you say "No" to more frequently? How?

*Developing communication skills is one of the most dramatic ways to differentiate yourself from others and set yourself on
a path to success. Protecting your single greatest asset is undoubtedly the most important. The next chapter shows
you the key to a sustainable, lucrative and enjoyable career.*

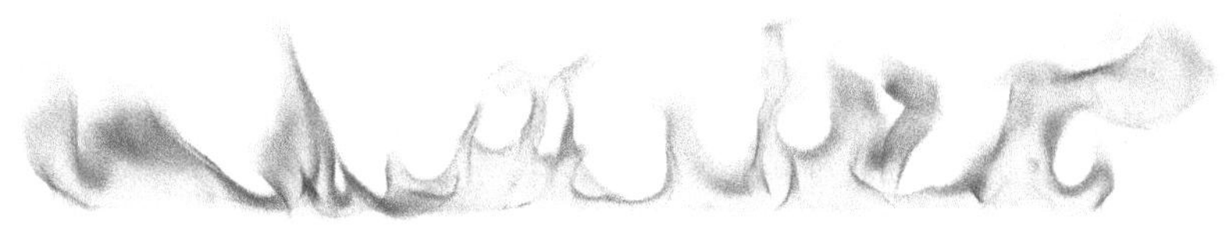

Chances are, you take your single greatest advantage for granted. This chapter offers minor lifestyle tweaks that will make your greatest asset work for, not against, you.

Essential Strategy #5:

Asset Protection

Shake Your Money Maker

WHAT DO YOU THINK IS your greatest professional asset? (Here's a hint: it's between your ears.)

Your brain's speed and capacity far exceeds any computer. Researchers in Japan recently tried to simulate the processing power of the brain. Using the 4th most powerful computer in the world, the "K Computer," they wired together almost 83,000 processors, which represents only 1 percent of the neurons your brain contains. Even with all that super-computer power, it took 40 minutes to replicate what the brain processes in 1 second.

That's right, 83,000 of the fastest processors in the world took 40 minutes to do what your brain does in 1 second.

One of your awesome brain's most awesome features is its plasticity, its malleability. A healthy brain continues to create new neural pathways and alter existing ones to accommodate learning, processing experiences, and forming memories, for your entire life.

Brain Plasticity Is Not Always Good

The distractions of the digital age are changing your brain. A recent study by Microsoft Corporation found that the digital lifestyle makes it difficult to stay focused. The human attention span shortened from 12 seconds to eight seconds since the year 2000. Humans now have a shorter attention span than a goldfish (nine seconds average). A separate 2014 British study found the average person shifts their attention between their smartphone, tablet and laptop 21 times in an hour.

This is bad news for anyone whose livelihood involves problem-solving or requires long periods of deep thought. Yeah, you.

However, it's good news for the smart career strategist who realizes developing their brain for deep thought increases their value, competitive edge, and career sustainability. Yeah, you!

Protect Your Asset

Weighing just three pounds and having the consistency of tofu, your brain is not necessarily an impressive organ. Although third in terms of size (after skin and liver), the brain hogs more energy than any other organ: 20–25 percent of the body's total load. What makes it special is its 100 billion neurons: specialized cells which transmit nerve impulses. Other cells live fairly short lives, but nerve cells live a long time—up to 100 years. In an adult, when neurons die because of disease or injury, they are not usually replaced.

The longevity of neurons makes their care more critical. Those cells will be around a while, subject to the conditions you create.

Care and Feeding of Your Brain

Your brain will happily serve you well until you're done with it, if you take care of it.

- **Hydrate** – Drink half your body weight in ounces, daily. Dehydration can impair short-term memory function, long-term memory recall, and immediate focus. A thirsty brain can cost you 10 IQ points.
- **Exercise** – Exercising the body is exercising the brain. Increasing blood flow in the brain's billions of capillaries removes toxins and provides oxygen and nutrients. Yummy!
- **Develop Digital Discipline** – Technology changes your brain. The same dopamine craving that creates heroin addiction draws you to look mindlessly at your nearest screen.
  - o Resist the siren call of technology when you're bored. Put the smart phone down!
  - o Set a schedule for checking email and stick to it.
  - o Use the web intentionally—no random surfing.
  - o Enjoy designated periods of time (evenings? weekends?) without technology.
  - o Protect the "margins" of your day. Avoid digital exposure during the first and last two hours of the day when your brain is most easily influenced.

o   Turn your phone screen to grayscale. This bypasses many of the brain's pleasure centers your phone is designed to activate.

- **Meditate** – MRI scans show that mediation increase gray matter concentration in the regions associated with memory, emotion regulation, and a sense of self and perspective taking. It improves concentration and attention, and reduces symptoms of depression, anxiety and pain. All that with no cost or side effects!

- **Minimize exposure to toxins** – the combination of longevity and sensitivity make brain cells particularly vulnerable to damage by free radicals and inflammation. It is in your brain's best interest—and, therefore, your own—to move in the direction of: limiting EMFs, avoiding sugar, managing stress, and avoiding known neurotoxins such as pesticides, lead, mercury, arsenic, fluoride, manganese, ethanol (drinking alcohol).

Undoing Damage

David Hendricks MD writes about growing the mind and healing the brain. Until 15 years ago we believed that the brain did not grow new neurons. There is an exception. We now know that the brain can grow new cells in the hippocampus, where damage occurs from childhood abuse, often leading to addiction and depression.

From brain scans we know areas of the brain work together to make positive emotions happen. We also know that trauma and abuse during childhood weaken precisely these areas of the brain. When we strengthen these areas during meditation, we are actually repairing the damages of childhood.

New neurons can be shaped by belief systems and meditation practices, making it possible for an abused, addicted or depressed person to eventually recover a perfectly healthy functioning brain.

Creating Circuitry

When you learn new information, form new beliefs, or create new habits, your brain "hard wires" the information by forming neural networks. Five factors influence the development of neural networks:

1. **Recency** – Recent associations are the strongest.
2. **Repetition** – Several exposures to new information are necessary.
3. **Multi-modality** – Involving the five senses (sight, sound, smell, touch, and taste) improves retention.
4. **Strong Emotion** – The more meaning you instill into a subject, the better you will engrain it.
5. **Unusualness** – Novel or rare experiences or information are retained better.

Take advantage of your brain's processing capability! Make your brain work for, not against, you. Program your brain with the following practices:

☐ **"Thumbs Up"** – Borrowed from Facebook (masters at algorithms that create dopamine compulsion), reinforce desired associations by pressing your built-in "Like" button. Consciously promote the selection of desired ideas in your consciousness.
   o Repeat helpful thought, silently or aloud.
   o Revisit or daydream about it.

- o Connect emotionally with gratitude or welcoming.
- o Reinforce with visual reminders.
- o Purposefully relax or allow yourself to feel good about the thought.
- ☐ **Mix it up** – Keep your brain guessing (and thereby, engaged) by doing things differently.
- ☐ **Affirmations** – consciously reprogram your brain with intentional statements that follow these guidelines:
  - o Positive wording
  - o Avoid "no" or "not"
  - o "I allow myself . . ."
  - o "I choose . . ."
  - o "I am . . ."
- ☐ **Fractals** – Whatever you focus on expands, repeats and displays at every scale. You see repeating patterns everywhere, because you've trained your brain to expect them. Expect positive and you'll see more of it.
- ☐ **"Eureka" Snap** – A finger snap to implant or cancel thoughts is effective because it involves 3 senses:
  - o Feeling pressure on finger
  - o Hearing happy little "pop" sound
  - o Seeing fingers with visual cortex (one of the largest, most powerful areas of brain)

Create ASSOCIATIONS by combining snap with word "cancel" and implanting replacement thought.

- ☐ **Use Intention** – the practice of taking a moment to consciously decide what you want to experience. Implement this as a habit with *Intentionology: 365 Days of Living on Purpose*, by this author (Available on Amazon)

- [ ] **Be true to your word** – Get your brain to trust you by consistently doing what you say you'll do (like leave work at 5, exercise at lunch, or learn Qi Gong).
- [ ] **Use Emotions** – You reprogram the unconscious majority of your brain best when you are in a very emotional state. Whatever you focus on and talk about with emotion, you get more of.
- [ ] **Repetition** – Study for short periods, walk away for regular 10-minute mind/body breaks, and then review 24 hours later, 1 week later and 6 months later for best retention.

Keep Learning

If you're not growing, you're dying. Beat burnout by continually reaching for the next thing, pushing your comfort zone, and raising your game. As a knowledge worker, you are not trading time for money. Knowledge is your currency, and a moving target. Keep up! Productivity as a knowledge worker is not just dependent on the time you give to work; it is also dependent on your energy and motivation, your ability to focus, your creativity and insight, and your raw intellectual power.

Self Coaching: Protect Your Asset

What sacrifices are you willing to make for your brain and why?

What sacrifices are off limits and why?

Continue the upward spiral. Reach for your tools, techniques, practices, strategies and support to keep yourself learning and growing. We need the gifts you came to bring!

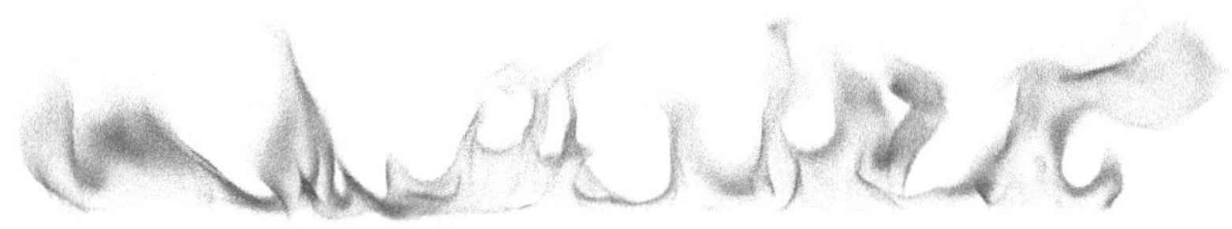

It Never Ends

I SHOULD HAVE WARNED YOU when you started this book, you can't unknow what you know.

You now know you're responsible for your success and happiness. You now know the full expression of True You is important and achievable. You now know you will need to use your tools today and every day for the rest of your life. You now know the power to change the direction of your life in a millisecond. This millisecond.

What are you going to do about it?

I can think of no other time in the history of mankind when it was so critical for each of us to bring our gifts to the planet. The world needs what you came to bring it.

You have a flame burning deep inside you. Stop reading and notice it now in the pit of your abdomen, just behind your navel. Is it a flicker or a roar? Does it fuel you, or threaten to consume you? Notice its qualities: longing or sated; eager or afraid; growing or dying?

Make friends with your flame. Revisit this book many times to evolve and refine how you nurture and protect it. In many ways, it's really all you have.

Also by This Author

Intentionology: 365 Days of Living On Purpose

Science says you can program your brain. Actually, you already have. The question is, how's that working for you?

Experience more of what you long for!

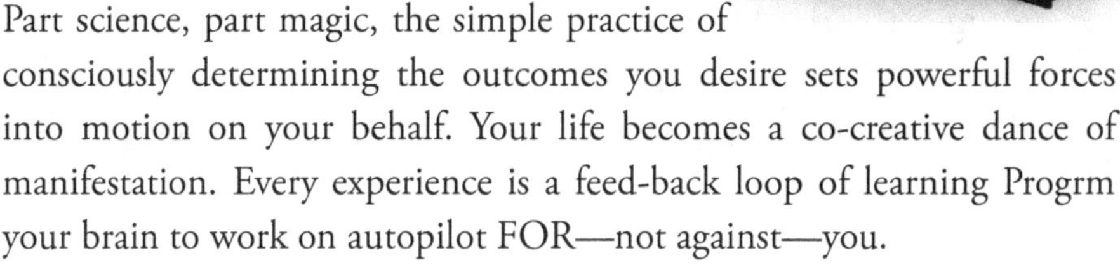

Part science, part magic, the simple practice of consciously determining the outcomes you desire sets powerful forces into motion on your behalf. Your life becomes a co-creative dance of manifestation. Every experience is a feed-back loop of learning Progrm your brain to work on autopilot FOR—not against—you.

This practical guide helps you develop a daily practice that replaces negative thought patterns with empowering, uplifting ones. A few minutes a day can change everything—forever—and it's FREE, easy, and life-changing. "Intenionology" serves you in mnay ways. Create a regular habit, or dip in and out as needed, or just enjoy beautiful inspriation when you necd it. Read for a quick shift.

You will develop a beautiful, meaningul, ever-evolving guide that will support you the rest of your life. 365 intentions for you to rewrite and reword, making them your own.

About the Author

E MPOWERMENT EXPERT, TRANSFORMATIONAL trainer, and whole-being, well-being whiz, Liz Garrett, is shifting lives with creative, reality-based programs that work on all levels–mind, body and spirit–for deep and lasting change in individuals and organizations. A successful business owner since 1998, and having worked collaboratively with execs for more than 20 years, she knows well the fire inside that either propels you to greatness, or consumes you in the effort. Find out more at www.LizGarrett.com.

Liz is Virginia born and raised, and still there. She prefers "y'all" for second-person plural, can slurp her weight in Chesapeake Bay oysters and, if she says to you, "Bless your heart," that's not necessarily a good thing.

Thank you for reading this book.

I appreciate your feedback and love hearing your thoughts, stories and experiences with the material, and suggestions for the next version.

Please leave a helpful review at Amazon.

Be sure to download your collateral resources at
https://trueyouadvantage.com/opposite/

Yours in wellness, purpose and abundance,

—Liz Garrett